OXFORD MEDICAL PUBLICATIONS

Talking to Cancer Patients
and Their Relatives

Talking to Cancer Patients and Their Relatives

ANN FAULKNER
Honorary Professor of Communications in Health Care,
University of Sheffield Medical School
Consultant and freelance lecturer
Education consultant to Trent Palliative Care Centre, Sheffield

PETER MAGUIRE
Director, Cancer Research Campaign Psychological Medicine Group,
and Honorary Consultant Psychiatrist, Christie Hospital,
Manchester

Oxford • New York • Tokyo
OXFORD UNIVERSITY PRESS

Oxford University Press, Walton Street, Oxford OX2 6DP
Oxford New York
Athens Auckland Bangkok Bogota Bombay
Buenos Aires Calcutta Cape Town Dar es Salaam
Delhi Florence Hong Kong Istanbul Karachi
Kuala Lumpur Madras Madrid Melbourne
Mexico City Nairobi Paris Singapore
Taipei Tokyo Toronto
and associated companies in
Berlin Ibadan

Oxford is a trade mark of Oxford University Press

Published in the United States by
Oxford University Press Inc., New York

A catalogue record for this book is available from the British Library

Library of Congress Cataloging in Publication Data
Faulkner, Ann.
Talking to cancer patients and their relatives/Ann Faulkner.
Peter Maguire.
(Oxford medical publications)
Includes index.
1. Cancer—Patients. 2. Medical personnel and patient.
I. Maguire, Peter. II. Title. III. Series.
RC262.F38 1994   616.99'4023—dc20   94–27387
ISBN 0 19 261605 6 (Pbk)

Typeset by Advance Typesetting Limited, Oxfordshire
Printed in Great Britain by Biddles Ltd, Guildford and King's Lynn

PREFACE

The diagnosis and treatment of cancer can cause major problems for patients and their relatives as they try to adapt to a fear-provoking diagnosis and an uncertain future. Effective communications between health professionals and patients, and their relatives, can play an important part in facilitating this adaptation. Doctors, nurses, and other workers in cancer care are increasingly aware of the need to improve their ability to interact effectively with patients, relatives, and colleagues.

The book is based on our research findings over a number of years with doctors, nurses, social workers, and members of the clergy. We are grateful to them for their willingness to have their skills scrutinized both before and after tuition.

The content of the book has been much influenced by our experience of running workshops and other courses. These have been based on our belief that assessment of problems is a crucial first step in delivering a high level of patient care, and our matching belief that the emotional survival of the health professional demands equal attention.

Our workshops have been based on the expressed needs of the participants for help with assessment of patients' and relatives' concerns, and the handling of difficult situations. We offer practical guidelines which have been tested at the 'sharp end' of clinical practice over many years, and which have been validated by those using them. Validation from patients and relatives has been especially important to us.

Finally, we make no apology for our pragmatic approach in our writing. We have included references where appropriate, and a resource list which we hope will cover related areas; but our focus has been on skills and strategies, and on describing a model of assessment which we have refined over a number of years.

A.F.
August 1994   P.M.

ACKNOWLEDGEMENTS

We would like to acknowledge those who have helped and encouraged us to develop our teaching of communication skills in the context of cancer care and to evaluate the impact of our methods.

The support of the Extra-Mural Department of the University of Manchester allowed us to develop our three-day workshops, while Help the Hospices have subsidized our multi-disciplinary five-day workshops in both interviewing and assessment skills and in teaching methods, which continue to be over-subscribed.

The Cancer Research Campaign funded our large evaluation programme, which has validated our teaching methods and allowed us to assess the impact of our teaching on the participants' skills, both in the short and longer term.

We have been particularly encouraged to continue this work because of the consistently positive feedback and constructive suggestions from the health professionals on our courses. We would particularly like to thank the Reverend Mo Witcombe for her advice on the chapter on spiritual issues.

Our long-suffering secretaries, Barbara Grimbley, Catherine Leslie, and Sue Moore, have our many thanks for their patience and co-operation in helping to produce the final manuscript.

Finally, we appreciate the love and support of our families and friends.

CONTENTS

1

Psychological morbidity: its recognition and management

The need to improve assessment skills: introduction
The diagnosis and treatment of cancer is associated with a substantial social and psychological morbidity (Derogatis *et al.* 1983; Greer 1985). Unfortunately, this morbidity often remains unrecognized and unresolved (Maguire 1992). Patients and their relatives are reluctant to disclose any problems, while health professionals are loath to enquire actively about them. This chapter will review the nature and extent of this morbidity and discuss the reasons why it remains undetected and unresolved.

Psychological morbidity
Psychological morbidity, in the form of an anxiety state, a depressive illness, or a combination of these, is more likely to develop if the patient who is newly diagnosed as having cancer is unable to surmount certain key psychological hurdles. These include:

1. *Uncertainty about the future.* Patients with cancer are faced with inevitable uncertainty about whether the cancer will recur and cause premature death. Any new physical symptoms may be perceived as a possible recurrence and heighten anxiety. Such fears will also be triggered by television programmes or articles in newspapers about cancer, and whenever patients attend a clinic for a follow-up appointment. While most can put the fear of recurrence to the back of their minds, some become plagued by it, and find they cannot stop thinking about it.

2. *The search for meaning.* When people are faced with adversity they cope with it better if they can find an acceptable explanation. Thus, a cancer patient will commonly ask 'Why me?', 'Why now?', or 'What have I done to bring this on?' Unfortunately, in the case of most cancers there are few clear risk factors apart from smoking. This leaves a vacuum into which patients can project their own ideas. Such ideas commonly involve either implicating their own personality, in the sense of their own perceived inability to express emotions like anger or to cope with stressful life events (particularly the breakdown of personal relationships or bereavement), or else blaming other people because they caused the stress. The danger with these theories is that people may become either obsessed with the idea that they caused their own cancer or bitter because they believe that other people brought it about.

3. Loss of control. Patients adapt more easily if they feel there is something they can contribute to the outcome of their illness. With an illness like coronary heart disease patients can try to modify their diet, weight, and level of exercise. Patients with cancer have no such factors they can easily modify, although some turn to psychological methods such as relaxation, visualization, or joining self-help groups. Patients who take constructive action to improve their outcomes adapt much better than do those who feel there is nothing they can do, and so feel increasingly helpless. Helplessness is associated with a strong risk of later depressive illness (Maguire 1992).

4. The need for openness. A major issue for cancer patients is whether to be open about their disease and treatment with friends, relatives, and employers. If they feel cancer has stigmatized them then they will be less likely to be open. They may also be secretive because they do not wish to cause upset to loved ones. Such secrecy hinders psychological adaptation. In contrast, openness allows patients to receive the necessary emotional and practical support.

Feelings of stigma, of feeling 'dirty', 'unclean', or 'contagious', can be intensified if cancer patients perceive that other people are withdrawing from them. Studies (Comaroff and Maguire 1981) have shown that some relatives and friends find it hard to maintain the same level of contact after a cancer diagnosis, because they are uneasy about what to say in conversation and frightened of upsetting the patient or the relatives, or of hearing bad news.

5. The need for emotional support. A key issue is whether patients perceive that they are getting adequate emotional support from friends and relatives (Harrison and Maguire 1993). Those who perceive that others care cope much better than those who feel that people around them do not understand their predicament.

Table 1.1 Symptoms of anxiety

Core mood disturbance	Key symptoms
Persistently tense, on edge, or unable to relax	Initial insomnia
	Irritability
Significantly more so than normal mood variation	Sweating, tremor, nausea
Cannot distract self or be distracted out of it	Poor concentration
	Indecisiveness
	Spontaneous panics

6. The need for medical support. Some cancer patients seek support readily from the general practitioner or hospital doctor, particularly when they meet a crisis. Others hold back because they do not wish to burden the doctor. There is then a danger of their need for support falling between the twin stools of the cancer centre and the general practitioner, with the consequence that they receive inadequate overall support. Doctors may play a part in this, particularly if the patient is experiencing a stormy illness which is not responding well to treatment. There is then a risk that the health professionals will withdraw, leaving the patient and family even more isolated.

As a general rule any patient who fails to surmount one or more of these hurdles is likely to develop an anxiety state, a depressive illness, or combination of the two within the first year of diagnosis, quite apart from any additional problems created by the cancer treatment itself.

Anxiety states
Anxious mood should be diagnosed when patients complain of a persistent inability to relax or stop worrying and are unable to distract themselves from these worries or be distracted by others, and this represents a significant change both quantitively and qualitatively from the patient's normal mood. For an anxiety state to be diagnosed there must be at least four or more other symptoms (Table 1.1), which may include: an inability to get off to sleep (initial insomnia); irritability; sweating, tremor, or nausea; impaired concentration; indecisiveness; and spontaneous panic attacks. Patients with this generalized anxiety disorder may also have irrational fears of specific situations, such as

Table 1.2 Symptoms of depression

Core mood disturbance	Key symptoms
Persistent low mood and/or inability to enjoy self	Repeated or early waking, excessive sleep
Significantly lower mood than normal variation	Irritability
Cannot snap out of it or be pulled out of it by others	Poor concentration
	Agitation or retardation
	Social withdrawal
	Negative self-ideation (e.g. hopeless, worthless, a burden)
	Diurnal variation of mood

meeting groups of people (social phobia) or leaving the house alone (agoraphobia).

Depressive illness
Depressed mood should be diagnosed when a patient complains of persistent low mood lasting at least two to four weeks that occupies over 50 per cent of the waking time. This lowering of mood should be significantly greater both quantitively and qualitatively than the patient's normal mood fluctuations. Patients must be unable to get out of this depression by their own efforts or to be distracted out of it by others.

A depressive illness should be diagnosed when the mood disturbance is accompanied by four or more other symptoms (Table 1.2), which may include: sleep disturbance (waking repeatedly in the night or waking early in the morning and being unable to get back to sleep) or excessive sleep; irritability; impairment of attention and concentration; agitation or retardation; loss of energy; social withdrawal; negative ideation (ideas of hopelessness, self-blame, guilt, worthlessness, feeling a burden, seeing no future, seeing life as pointless); suicidal ideas; diurnal variation of mood (where the patient experiences significant lowering of mood at a particular time of day); loss of appetite or weight; and constipation.

In making a diagnosis, allowance should be made for the possibility that physical symptoms like loss of energy, appetite, and weight could be due to the progression of the cancer or its recurrence. So particular attention should be paid to the patient's mood, current ideas, and thinking. A common error is to regard depression in cancer patients as understandable, and to argue that treatment is unnecessary. This is analogous to withholding analgesia and not setting a fracture following a bad fall, on the grounds that the pain and fracture are understandable consequences of the fall.

Adjustment disorder
Sometimes, patients have either anxious mood, or depressed mood, or both, but too few other symptoms to be diagnosed as having an anxiety state or a depressive illness. In this case they are regarded as having an adjustment disorder, in which they are reacting in an exaggerated way to a known stressor, i.e. the cancer.

The effects of cancer treatments
Surgery—the loss of a body part
Surgery may involve the removal of a body part, such as a breast or limb. Patients then have to try to adapt to a change in body image, which will be difficult if that body part was important to their sense of psychological well-being. For example, up to 25 per cent of women fail to adapt to the loss of a breast, despite being given an adequate external breast prosthesis (Maguire *et al.* 1983). Three types of body image may develop. First, the patient may be unable to accept that she is no longer whole. This loss of physical integrity can make her feel increasingly vulnerable psychologically, and more likely to fail to adapt to any other similar stressful events. Second, she may feel a heightened sense of self-consciousness, and worry that people can somehow tell that she has lost a breast, even when she takes steps to conceal her shape. Finally, some women feel much less attractive and feminine, and come to believe that their partners can no longer accept them.

Continued inability to adapt to the loss of a body part, regardless of the part involved, is highly predictive of subsequent anxiety, depression, and sexual difficulties.

Surgery—loss of a body function
The fashioning of a stoma after resection of an anorectal cancer is a good example of the way in which treatment of cancer may result in

the loss of an important bodily function. Other examples include loss of speech after laryngectomy and loss of fertility following hysterectomy or oophorectomy after the treatment of gynaecological cancers.

Up to a third of patients who have a stoma formed after resection of cancer of the bowel become clinically anxious and/or depressed (Thomas *et al.* 1987). There may be two problems causing this mood disturbance. First, they may be unable to tolerate the stoma because it represents an 'obscene' part of themselves. Alternatively, their concerns may centre on managing the bag. They may fear that the bag will bulge, leak, smell, burst, or make a noise, and so interfere seriously with personal relationships and sexuality. Indeed, some individuals become so fearful that they will not leave the security of their own home in order to avoid embarrassment. Others only venture outside when they have mapped out the position of public toilets and know where to go if there is a problem with the bag. Similarly, patients may avoid going on holiday because of worry about the effect of change on diet or the problems of gaining access to toilets.

Those who have yet to form an intimate relationship face the particular dilemma about the point at which they should mention their stoma to a potential partner. Fears associated with the bag and of rejection may contribute to the development of sexual difficulties, though these may also have an organic component. For surgery can result in destruction of the nerve supply to the genital organs.

Women who undergo gynaecological surgery face the loss of fertility (Corney *et al.* 1992). This may exacerbate feelings of losing control of oneself and one's bodily functions, and may also exacerbate any body-image problems.

Radiotherapy

Radiotherapy commonly causes fatigue and sore skin. Other side-effects depend on the area irradiated. There is a strong relationship between the development of adverse effects during radiotherapy and subsequent anxiety and depression (Devlen *et al.* 1987). Radiotherapy may also promote anxiety because patients fear that they are only having radiotherapy because some cancer cells must have been left behind after surgery.

Chemotherapy

Chemotherapy, especially in combination, can increase the risk of anxiety and depression. As with radiotherapy, there is a strong relationship between the development of adverse side-effects, particularly nausea, vomiting, and diarrhoea, and the risk of anxiety and depression (Devlen *et al.* 1987).

Conditioned nausea and vomiting occur in up to 25 per cent of patients (Morrow 1982), and are likely to provoke anxiety and depression. Characteristically, a patient experiences nausea and vomiting during the first or second course of treatment. The patient then finds that any sound, sight, or smell which reminds him or her of treatment provokes the same side-effects reflexively. This can lead to a phobic reaction, and ultimately to dropping out of treatment.

Sexual problems also result because chemotherapy lowers the production of the hormones that are necessary for promoting fertility. While men can now bank their sperm in advance of chemotherapy, there is no similar technology available to store women's ova. And while some women may be able to have hormone replacement therapy to prevent menopausal symptoms, this is contraindicated in breast cancer.

Other treatments
Early studies, for example in respect of bone-marrow transplantation, have suggested that fears about treatment-related mortality, concerns about the donor, and the experiencing of prolonged isolation increase psychiatric morbidity in the short and longer term (Andrykowski *et al.* 1989).

Organic factors
When patients with cancer present with an anxiety state or depressive illness or adjustment disorder it is important to remember there may be underlying organic factors which are contributing to their development. These include an occult recurrence of the cancer, the use of particular drugs like steroids in high doses, biochemical changes like the raised calcium associated with advanced breast cancer, or direct effects of chemotherapy on the brain. It is also important to note that cancer can cause organic mental disorders in a minority of patients.

Organic confusional states
These often have a sudden onset, and there is usually a fluctuation in the level of the patient's consciousness. This is evident in their being disorientated to time and place and in an impairment of their concentration. These symptoms may be worse at night. However,

fluctuations can be rapid, with changes being noted from minute to minute or hour to hour. These patients usually experience perceptual abnormalities. These may take the form of illusions where the person is misperceived as someone else or some other object. The perceptional abnormalities may be more serious and may include hallucinations (both auditory and visual), and there may be paranoid ideation where patients begin to fear that the nursing and medical staff are out to harm them. Confusional states are often accompanied by changes in mood, including fear and irritability. There may be abnormalities of behaviour, including plucking of the bedclothes, over-activity, or inertia.

There are many possible causes of confusional states in cancer patients. Metabolic changes due to cancer or the drugs used for treatment are especially important. You should therefore check if a new drug has been started and whether there has been any change in the underlying biochemistry and haematology.

The development of confusional states should also alert the health professional to the possibility of alcohol or drug misuse.

There are several reasons why alcohol abuse is associated with cancer. Firstly, it may be because the patient has found it difficult to adapt to the hurdles discussed at the beginning of this chapter. Second, it may be an attempt to relieve the suffering and torment caused by the development of an anxiety state or depressive illness. Finally, alcoholics are at high risk of developing cancer of the oesophagus, stomach, and pancreas.

Dementia

Dementia refers to a gradual deterioration in the intellect, personality, and behaviour in a setting of clear consciousness. Most cases are irreversible, but a small proportion are reversible (including dementias due to a vitamin B_{12} deficiency, hypothyroidism, and subdural haematomas). The two commonest causes of dementia are Alzheimer's disease and multiple infarcts. Both are generally seen in patients above the age of 70 years. Dementia in cancer patients may result from cerebral metastases.

Behavioural problems in children

Behavioural problems are common in children with cancer. These include temper tantrums, bed-wetting, soiling, and excessive clinging and dependency (Peck 1979). Some children appear to develop personality problems in later life. Psychiatric problems are also far commoner in the physically healthy siblings of cancer patients, illustrating how a serious illness such as cancer affects the whole family. Some problems in the siblings are due to their being spoiled or over-protected by parents and relatives.

Children who have survived the diagnosis and treatment of cancer have been shown to have cognitive deficits and learning difficulties. The long-term outcome of these remain to be determined, as does the question of the extent to which adults are susceptible to such organic change. Two theories have been proposed. First, they may be a direct result of the effects of chemotherapy or radiotherapy on the brain. Secondly, cancer treatment may cause a period of immunosuppression which allows viral infection of the brain to occur, leading to subsequent cognitive impairment. Learning difficulties, whatever their cause, tend to be exacerbated, as children with cancer often have long periods of absence from school.

Social morbidity
While the stress of cancer and cancer treatment brings many families closer together it can also drive families apart, particularly when there are pre-existing problems within key relationships. This is especially true in relation to childhood cancers (Faulkner *et al.* 1995).

It has also been noted that a significant minority of cancer patients fail to return to work even though they are deemed free of disease and are off treatment (Devlen *et al.* 1987). This can be due to patients' making a positive reappraisal of their goals in life. In other patients it may represent 'illness behaviour', that is, they are getting some clear gain from maintaining their symptoms even though they are free of disease and off treatment.

Some cancer patients find themselves stigmatized when they attempt to return to work. They are either not re-employed or are offered a job at a much lower level than before.

Some patients may experience a stormy illness and require a considerable amount of treatment. The time taken off work may result in severe financial difficulties and increased stress within the family.

It can also result in a loss of role, so that a person who was formerly the hub of the family begins to feel angry and resentful that he is no longer able to fulfil his role and yet cannot adapt to the inevitable change. This will make it difficult for him and his family to adapt to the cancer and the treatment.

Hidden morbidity

Although it has been established that psychosocial morbidity is common in cancer patients and their relatives it is usually recognized and treated appropriately in only 15 to 25 per cent of cases (Maguire 1992). So, the reasons for this low rate of detection need to be considered.

Reasons for low detection rate

Both patients and their relatives and health professionals contribute to this.

Patients wrongly believe that these adverse effects of diagnosis and treatment are an inevitable consequence of their disease. Consequently, there is no point in mentioning them. They also do not wish to appear a nuisance or inadequate, or to burden the health professional unnecessarily. They feel it is more legitimate to mention physical aspects than psychological and social issues. They believe this because they claim that they are not often asked questions by health professionals about these areas. Since the consultation is often short in duration they fear that less attention will be paid to their disease if they take up the time talking about psychological and social problems (Maguire 1985).

Paradoxically, the more patients come to like and respect health professionals the less likely they are to burden them with psychosocial problems, because they do not want to upset them or cause more difficulties than the health professions are already experiencing in trying to manage the situation. This is analogous to the way patients protect relatives from the reality of their suffering.

When patients disclose problems they are selective in what they disclose. Thus, they tend to tell the doctor or nurse only of physical problems, because they believe that is what the latter are concerned with, whereas with a psychiatrist or psychologist they tend to disclose only psychological problems. So it is difficult for a health professional to get a comprehensive picture of patients' problems unless patients are interviewed in the ways that are discussed in Chapters 3 and 4.

Health professionals contribute to this low detection rate in two ways. They avoid asking the kinds of questions that would indicate an interest in psychological and social problems. Secondly, they try to keep the patient at a safe emotional distance by either ignoring cues about psychological and social aspects, or avoiding clarifying them, or by trying to distance themselves from the patient's emotions and concerns by using strategies which are described in Chapter 2.

Reasons for these deficiencies

When health professionals who are experienced in cancer care were interviewed in depth and asked to consider why they failed to pick up important social and psychological problems in their patients, they readily admitted that they assumed that their patients would disclose spontaneously any such problems; hence, there was no need to go searching for them. However, they also admit that they are afraid of probing into social and psychological aspects because they fear opening a 'Pandora's box' and unleashing strong emotions like anger, despair, and hopelessness (Comaroff and Maguire 1981; Rosser and Maguire 1982). They are afraid of such emotions because they do not feel they have been equipped by their training to help patients handle these feelings. They believe it would take too much time within the consultation and prevent them carrying out their key task of ensuring the patient's physical survival.

They are especially afraid that if they do probe psychologically the patient will 'cave in' and not be able to cope. They are also worried that they will be asked difficult questions like 'How long have I got to live?' or 'Am I dying?', which they do not know how to handle. They are worried that they may get too close to the patient's real predicament and emotional distress, and that this will compromise their own personal survival. For example, it can be extremely hard for a nursing sister to talk to a woman of her own age who is dying of breast cancer and who has two young children at home without identifying with her and feeling extremely upset.

Getting in touch with patients' real predicaments will inevitably remind the health professional of the limitations of modern medicine. For it is not possible to cure many cancers, and a substantial number of patients still suffer and die from them. This can be especially hard to deal with if the health professionals are not seeing patients who have done well, as well as those who have relapsed or have developed terminal illness. This can lead them to question the value of medicine and their own worth (Rosser and Maguire 1982). There will then be a tendency for them to increase their use of distancing to avoid experiencing this self-doubt.

Even if health professionals are willing to probe there is then the problem of what they will do with the information. Unless they perceive that they will be supported in taking on a more psychological and social role, and have psychiatric back-up when they need to refer patients for more expert help, it is unlikely that they will risk exploring the patient's problems. This is particularly unfortunate since there are effective ways of treating the patient's psychological and social morbidity.

Management of psychosocial morbidity
Adjustment disorder
Treatment usually consists of short-term crisis-orientated psychotherapy. Clarification of the medical situation combined with regular reassurance and practical and emotional support will usually enable patients to recover and adapt to their situations. In severe cases it might be worth referring the patient to a Liaison Psychiatrist for advice on what might be the best course of action to take and whether they also need specific behavioural and cognitive strategies—for example, progressive muscular relaxation—to control symptoms of anxiety. Sometimes, there is a place for the short-term use of medication to relieve anxiety symptoms or to enable the patient to sleep. A one-week prescription of temazepam (10 to 20 mg at night) on an as-needed basis may suffice. Similarly, the prescription of diazepam 5 mg three times a day as needed to combat daytime anxiety may be initiated for a short period. If depressive symptoms are marked, though not sufficient to merit a diagnosis of depressive illness, it is often worth commencing an antidepressant. This can always be withdrawn later if patients make a rapid recovery from their adjustment disorder.

Anxiety state
If patients are unable to cope from day to day or comply with treatment for their cancers it is worth considering the use of an anxiolytic drug (such as diazepam) for two to three weeks initially, but no longer, because of the risk of dependence. It is important to advise the patient to take this only when necessary. Once there has been some alleviation of mood they should be helped to learn how to manage their anxiety using anxiety-management training (Jannoun et al. 1982). Anxiety-management training involves helping the patient learn progressive muscular relaxation and positive imaging. It may be necessary to refer the patient to a clinical psychologist for this, unless the health professional doing the assessment has been trained in the use of these techniques. If the anxiety is provoked by irrational fears of recurrence or concerns about body image then cognitive therapy has a place (Goddard 1982; Tarrier and Maguire 1984; Moorey 1991). Here the therapist critically analyses the antecedents of these irrational beliefs and their consequences, and then challenges them and suggests more appropriate thought processes.

If patients have strong conditioned responses prior to chemotherapy it is worth recommending they take lorazepam for two to three days before each infusion in a dose of 2 mg at a time up to three times a day.

Sometimes, these measures are insufficient to help the patient cope more effectively. It is, therefore, worth considering a major tranquillizer (like clopromazine) or a tricyclic antidepressant with sedative properties (like amitryptiline). When somatic symptoms predominate it is worth considering a beta-blocker like propanalol.

If the anxiety is fuelled by realistic concerns about prognosis then the guidelines given in the chapter on informing the patient about how to manage uncertainty should be followed.

Depressive illness

This should be treated promptly with antidepressant medication, which is effective in over 80 per cent of cancer patients, yet tolerable, with relatively few adverse effects. Appropriate drugs might include dothiepin (Prothiaden) or fluoxetine (Prozac). When treating patients with antidepressants it is important to make several points if they are to comply with treatment. First, they are given to correct a biochemical disturbance brought about by the stress of cancer or cancer treatment. Second, they do not cause physical or psychological dependence. Third, the drug will need to be taken for at least 4 to 6 months to prevent relapse. Fourth, the prescription of the drug is only the first step in helping the patient with additional complaints like body-image problems or fears of recurrence. Fifth, the antidepressant medication must be taken regularly as prescribed, and not just when the patient is feeling low. Finally, the patient should be informed that improvement will take at least 3 to 4 weeks to become apparent, and the drug should not be stopped in the mean time. However, should any untoward side-effects develop, the health professional should be alerted.

Body-image problems

Behavioural therapy helps many patients with body-image problems. Treatments include graded exposure to looking at the affected part after learning progressive relaxation. Alternatively, if the beliefs about body image are irrational, cognitive therapy may be tried. There may also be a place for surgical reconstruction, providing the patient has been properly informed about the pros and cons of the advised procedure.

Sexual problems

Sexual problems may be organic or psychological in aetiology. The mode of treatment will depend on a proper assessment of the contribution of these various factors. However, when the problems are primarily psychological conjoint marital therapy has an important place (Masters and Johnson 1970).

Training

Fortunately, experienced health professionals recognize that a major reason for their reluctance to enquire about social and psychological problems is that they feel they have had insufficient training in key assessment skills or in strategies that would allow them to deal with the difficult situations that crop up continually when they relate to cancer patients and their relatives. Thus, they will have had little systematic training in how to break bad news, to deal with anger, despair, and distress, to challenge denial, to break collusion, to help explore patients' body-image problems, sexual difficulties, anxiety, and depression, or to confront colleagues with whom they disagree about patient management (Maguire and Faulkner 1988). They are usually uncertain about the criteria they should use to determine whether or not to refer a patient for psychological or psychiatric help. This book aims to provide practical guidelines about how to carry out an assessment of cancer patients to determine their current problems, how to monitor their subsequent progress, how to handle the difficult situations that will be encountered, and how to communicate with patients in ways that will reduce the associated social, psychological, and psychiatric morbidity. It will also discuss methods of training that will help health professionals acquire the key skills and strategies.

Summary

The diagnosis and treatment of cancer is associated with a substantial social, psychological, and psychiatric morbidity. Effective treatments are available which can result in as many as 80 per cent of patients so affected making a full recovery. However, only 20 per cent of patients so affected are usually recognized as needing help. This is because most health professionals have not had the opportunity to acquire the necessary assessment and communication skills. These skills and strategies will be illustrated, and methods of training will be discussed.

References

Andrykowski, M. A., Henslee, P. J., and Farrall, M. G. (1989). Physical and psychosocial functioning of adult survivors of allogeneic bone marrow transplantation. *Bone Marrow Transplantation*, **4**, 75–81.

Comaroff, J. and Maguire, P. (1981). Ambiguity and the search for meaning: childhood leukaemia in the modern clinical context. *Social Science and Medicine*, **158**, 115–23.

Corney, R. H., Everett, H., Howells, A., and Crowther, M. E. (1992). Psychosocial adjustment following major gynaecological surgery for carcinoma of the cervix and vulva. *Journal of Psychosomatic Research*, **36**, 561–8.

Derogatis, L. R., Morrow, G. R., Fetting, J., Penman, D., Piasetsky, F., Schmale A. M., Henrichs, M., and Carnicke C. L. M. (1983). The prevalence of psychiatric disorders among cancer patients. *Journal of the Americal Medical Association*, **249**, 751–7.

Devlen, J., Maguire P., Phillips, P., Crowther, D., and Chambers H. (1987). Psychological problems associated with diagnosis and treatment of lymphomas. II: A prospective study. *British Medical Journal*, **295**, 956–7.

Faulkner, A., Pearce, G., and O'Keeffe, C. (1995). *When a child has cancer*. Chapman and Hall, London. (In Press.)

Goddard, A. (1982). Cognitive behaviour therapy and depression. *British Journal of Hospital Medicine*, **27**, 248–50.

Greer, S. (1985). Cancer: psychiatric aspects. In *Recent advances in clinical psychiatry: 5* (ed. K. Granville-Grossman), pp. 87–104. Churchill Livingstone, Edinburgh.

Harrison, J. and Maguire, P. (1994). Predictors of psychiatric morbidity in cancer patients. *British Journal of Psychiatry*. (In Press.)

Jannoun, L., Oppenheimer, C., and Gelder, M. (1982). A self-help treatment programme for anxiety state patients. *Behavioural Therapy*, **13**, 103–11.

Maguire, P. (1985). Barriers to psychological care of the dying. *British Medical Journal*, **291**, 1711–13.

Maguire, P. (1992). Improving the recognition and treatment of affective disorders in cancer patients. In *Recent advances in psychiatry, 7* (ed. K. Granville-Grossman), pp. 15–30. Churchill Livingstone, Edinburgh.

Maguire, P. and Faulkner, A. (1988). How to do it: improve the counselling skills of doctors and nurses in cancer care. *British Medical Journal*, **197**, 847–9.

Maguire, P., Brooke, M., Tait, A., Thomas, C., and Sellwood, R. A. (1983). The effect of counselling on physical disability and social recovery after mastectomy. *Clinical Oncology*, **9**, 319–24.

Masters, W. H. and Johnson, V. E. (1970). *Human sexual inadequacy*. Churchill, London.

Moorey, S. (1991). Cognitive behaviour therapy. *Hospital Update*, September, 726–32.

Morrow, G. R. (1982). Prevalence and correlates of anticipatory nausea and vomiting in chemotherapy patients. *Journal of National Cancer Institute*, **68**(1), (April 1982), 585–8.

Peck, B. (1979). Effects of childhood cancer on long term survivors and their families. *British Medical Journal*, **1**, **6155**, 1327–9.

Rosser, J. E. and Maguire, P. (1982). Dilemmas in general practice: the care of the cancer patient. *Social Science and Medicine*, **16**, 315–22.

Tarrier, N. and Maguire, P. (1984). Treatment of psychological distress following mastectomy: an initial report. *Behaviour Research and Therapy*, **22**, 81–4.

Thomas, C., Madden, F., and Jehu, D. (1987). Psychological effects of stomas—on psychosocial morbidity one year after surgery. *Journal of Psychosomatic Research*, **31**, 311–16.

2

'Distancing' by health professionals

Caring for patients and their families when there is a diagnosis such as cancer, and/or a poor prognosis, is not easy. The work is often emotionally charged, and the health professional may have to answer awkward and challenging questions, for example 'Am I dying?', 'Can't they find a cure?'; deal with difficult situations, for instance collusion; and risk becoming involved in painful issues and decisions. These situations will be discussed in Chapter 7.

A common response to difficulties is for health professionals to distance themselves from patients and relatives. This has the effect of saving the health professional from some of the stress of caring, but may mean that the patients' real needs and morbidity remain unrecognized. Many cancer nurses feel that they should not be stressed by caring for patients; but this raises many questions, not least about the mechanisms that are used to avoid the pain of patients and relatives who are attempting to come to grips with a severe life crisis. Maguire and Faulkner, in evaluating workshops to help health professionals improve their communication skills, found a high level of 'blocking' among participants on the courses. If health professionals are accurately to assess and meet patients' needs, distancing techniques need to be recognized for what they are, so that insight may be gained into 'why' and 'how' distancing can happen. If professionals learn to open themselves to their patients' reality, they will need to consider the cost to themselves. This raises the important issue of survival, which will be addressed in Chapter 12 of this book.

Neutral material
There is a well-held belief that, in order to gain a patient's trust, some 'relationship-building' must take place before the patient's problems are mentioned. Much time may be spent in encouraging a patient to talk about her home, the weather, her taste in TV programmes, or other

'neutral' topics, when what the patient needs is permission to talk about her current concerns. If the patient tries to 'home in' on more pressing matters she is often blocked, and may then feel unable to disclose her worries. Consider the following conversation in terms of neutral materials versus patients' concerns:

Nurse:	Hello, Mr Wright; you found the ward, then?
Mr Wright:	Yes, but ...
Nurse:	It's an old hospital, this. All corridors, and easy to get lost.
Mr Wright:	I could do with being lost!
Nurse:	Don't say that. I see from your notes that you have come quite a long way. At least the weather is lovely just now.
Mr Wright:	Yes.
Nurse:	And you *are* brown. Do you have a garden?

In the above sequence the nurse is using neutral material to an extent that she blocks the patient when he gives cues that he has other concerns, for instance 'I could do with being lost'. This has the effect of distancing on two counts. First, the talk of the hospital and the weather means that patient's concerns are at least delayed. Second, and perhaps more important, is the fact that the patient is learning to follow the nurse's lead and realize that she does not want to hear of real problems. Faulkner and Maguire (1984) found that most conversations between nurses and cancer patients followed this neutral pattern.

Ignoring cues
In the above sequence, the patient gave the important cue 'I could do with being lost!' One cannot assume a knowledge of why the patient wants to be lost; but it is reasonable to suggest that, had the nurse explored this cue, she would have been at risk of getting into potentially painful areas with the patient:

Nurse:	Hello, Mr Wright, you found the ward then?
Mr Wright:	Yes, but ...
Nurse:	It's an old hospital, this. All corridors and easy to get lost.
Mr Wright:	I could do with being lost!
Nurse:	What makes you say that?
Mr Wright:	Well, it's all a bit of a mess. I've been told I have to have this treatment; but I'll be sick, won't I, and they won't even promise that it will work!

In the above sequence, the nurse very quickly identifies two major issues for the patient which she may find very painful—i.e. the effect of aggressive treatment and the uncertainty of the patient's future.

Ignoring cues as a way of maintaining distance is both common and effective, because often the topic which the patient wishes to raise may be seen to be socially unacceptable. In our culture, many topics are seen to be 'taboo', and these generally include health concerns. If the health professional ignores the cue several times, the patient may still continue to attempt to talk about his concern. However, if the cue is repeatedly ignored, the patient will eventually be educated that it is not appropriate to raise emotional concerns. It takes a really assertive patient to continue to offer the cue after a few tries, or to make his or her concern more precise, but even then the nurse or doctor can maintain his or her distance as follows:

Doctor: Well Dorothy, I expect you will be glad to get this operation over.

Dorothy: It's not the operation ... [cue].

Doctor: You'll have a little injection, and next thing you will be back in your own bed.

Dorothy: But it's the thought of the stoma ... [more explicit cue].

Doctor: And after a day or so the specialist nurse will show you just how easy it is.

In this sequence, the doctor ignored the patient's cues and continued to give information about the operation. With a major concern about the reality of a stoma on her mind it is unlikely that Dorothy would absorb the information being offered.

From the growing literature on ignored or missed cues, there has arisen a belief that each cue should be picked up when it is offered; but of course this is unrealistic. Most of us miss cues from time to time; but patients will usually offer again, and only give up trying when they sense the professional's reluctance to respond to their concerns.

Selective attention to cues

Most patients have a number of concerns when they are facing severe illness or impending death. These may range from practical matters to physical and emotional problems, and all may be offered as cues, with some patients giving several cues at once. For example:

Jack: Oh, its all such a mess—I wanted things to be special for Judy, but now I'm so ill it's all fallen on her, and

	I'm not sure she wants to look after me—or if we can afford for her to stay at home. My pension won't go far on its own.
Doctor:	We can get the social worker to talk to you about your financial problems.

In the above disclosure Jack raised several issues. He gave a cue that suggested that he might be feeling that he had failed Judy. Other cues suggested that she may be overloaded and that she may not want to care for him; and one raised the practical matter of financial difficulties. The doctor selected the practical cue; but a skilled professional would summarize all the concerns, and then follow the patient's lead on priorities. In picking up the cue on practical matters, which are more readily soluble than the emotional concerns, the doctor maintains his distance. This focus will mean that Jack's feelings may not be assessed, and other psychological issues may also be ignored.

Inappropriate encouragement

One very potent distancing tactic is the use of inappropriate encouragement, where the patient's concerns are trivialized in the course of encouraging him or her to think positively. The doctor, for example, who missed Dorothy's concerns on having a stoma, encouraged her by saying 'The specialist nurse will show you how easy it is! Come on, cheer up, I know of many famous people who have stomas.'

In these situations, the patient's fears and worries do not go away; but individual patients may begin to worry that perhaps something is wrong with *them*—that *they* are silly, inept, and in some way wrong to be reacting so badly to their current predicament. This distancing tactic will almost certainly cause the patients to stop articulating their concerns, and may also lead to damage to the patient's self-image, or anger directed towards the enormous difficulty of adjusting to a life crisis.

Dorothy, for example, could not respond to the notion that caring for her stoma would be easy, because she found the whole idea totally revolting, and was unable even to begin to think of looking at or touching her stoma. Even worse was the thought of others seeing her 'disfigurement'.

Inappropriate encouragement can also be used by underlining the individual's responsibility to others. Let us stay with Dorothy, who did not respond to the first encouragement and now has the added worry that she is somehow at fault for being unable to cope.

Nurse:	Come on Dorothy, still down in the dumps?
Dorothy:	Well, it's hardly a cheerful outlook.

Nurse: Oh, do cheer up, others manage! And you owe it to your family to get to grips with it—not very nice for them when they visit—don't want Hubby more worried, do we?

The above encouragement, again, did not take Dorothy's worries away, but added to her burden of guilt and anger by implying that her reactions were selfish. If worried relatives are also encouraged to be cheerful for the sake of the patient, an enormous barrier can be erected, which may well lead to collusion (see Chaper 7).

Inappropriate encouragement is often accompanied by premature, or false, reassurance.

Premature reassurance

Premature reassurance is given *before* all the patient's key problems have been elicited, often in an attempt to cheer the patient or encourage more positive attitudes towards disease or prognosis. The difficulty is that subsequent events may reveal the reassurance to be inappropriate to the individual, and in fact inaccurate. For this reason, all key problems should be elicited and priorities identified. For example, when Jack was worried that Judy did not really want to look after him, it would be very tempting for the health professional to reply on the lines of 'of course she wants to look after you, she hasn't stopped loving you just because you are ill!' Such reassurance is not only premature, in that we don't know all the problems *or* how Judy feels; but it is also presumptuous, in that quite large assumptions are being made about the couple's relationship.

Premature reassurance of this sort has two functions for the heath professional—firstly, it gives the satisfaction of meeting the patient's need to be reassured; but more importantly, it does so without the professional becoming intimately involved in the emotional concerns of the patient. If, for example, instead of premature reassurance, the professional had offered to talk to Judy, the result might not have been easy to manage. For example:

Nurse: [after introduction] Judy, I wanted a word with you, because Jack is anxious about dying at home.

Judy: But he is determined that that is what he wants to do.

Nurse: And you?

Judy: I have to go along with it. I'm his wife—it's the least he can expect.

Nurse: You say you *have* to go along with it—how do *you* feel about it?

Judy:	I'm scared.
Nurse:	Scared?
Judy:	I don't know anything about dying. I'll probably exasperate him—he isn't easy when he is well; and what if I wake up and find him dead? Oh God, NO— I wish he would stay here, where I can just about cope!

The professional is now in the painful arena of handling two people with differing needs, for whom where may not be a happy solution. Distancing allows the health professional to soften a situation and avoid facing the reality.

False reassurance

It is this need to have seemingly positive outcomes which leads health carers to give false reassurance rather than confront a reality which could be painful. Its use allows distancing in the name of protecting the patient from information which may be damaging. It happens particularly in situations where either the doctor or a relative is colluding over the patient's diagnosis and/or prognosis (Chapter 7).

Fred Senior had come into hospital for investigations, to be found to have cancer of the bowel with metastatic spread. His prognosis was poor; but when he asked the nurse about his tests she felt that she could not upset him. This was partly out of concern for Fred, but also because she did not feel able to deal with his distress.

The exchange went as follows:

Fred:	Nurse! The doctor said my tests would be back today, and they would have looked at the X-rays.
Nurse:	That's right. They will come and talk to you soon.
Fred:	Can't you tell me?
Nurse:	[hesitant] I'm not too good at X-rays yet.
Fred:	But they said it would come with a report! You've seen that, haven't you?
Nurse:	Yes, and you are not to worry. The doctors will soon fix you up and have you a different man.
Fred:	I wish I could believe it.
Nurse:	You *must* believe it—the doctors are very good here.

In the above exchange, the nurse felt that she had tried to soften the situation and to get Fred thinking in a positive manner without herself getting involved in painful emotional reactions. Other ways to avoid answering difficult questions are to switch the topic or focus of the interaction.

Switching the topic

There will be few of us who have not used, or encountered, the strategy of changing the subject. When we hear or use the strategy, the message is a clear 'back off please, I don't wish to discuss this'. It is a form of social control which allows an individual to raise a subject, and to drop it if it is unacceptable. We may hear that a friend is getting divorced, but not know how painful she finds the subject. We might say 'I'm sorry, Mary, to hear things haven't worked out for you', and if she replies 'What do you think of all this fuss over our pay increase?', we accept that Mary does not want to talk about her divorce at the moment.

Professionals switch topics for the same reasons—that they do not wish to pursue a topic, answer a question, or get involved in a particular issue. The patient, who has learned from his own social experience, will know that discussion of his concern is not acceptable. As with giving cues, he may try again, but may evenually accept that the health professional does not wish to hear of his concerns. Fred, for example, was eventually told by the doctor that his bowel was 'a bit cancerous', and could not understand why he was not offered an operation.

Fred:	My cousin had this sort of bowel trouble—he had to have a colostomy.
Nurse:	I've got the menus here, do you want fish or meat pie?
Fred:	Oh, the fish. But nurse, why did my cousin have an operation—I'm sure it's the same sort of trouble.
Nurse:	Do you come from a big family?
Fred:	Well, I have one brother and two cousins. We all lived near when we were kids.
Nurse:	And you still keep in touch?
Fred:	My cousin …
Nurse:	I must go: I have the rest of the menus to do.

Fred learned that trying to make sense of a serious disease without the offer of an operation was an unacceptable topic to the nurse; but he continued to worry, and his concerns were greater in that he interpreted the nurse's reluctance to talk as a cue that his situation was too serious to be disclosed.

Switching the focus to relatives

Switching the focus of an interview is a more subtle form of distancing, because the interaction continues to flow smoothly. Fred was aware that the menus were a 'Please change the subject' ploy, and his later mention of his cousin also provoked the nurse's invoking the menus as an excuse to leave. Consider the following interaction:

Jack:	Oh, it's such a mess, and I wanted it to be special for Judy, but now I'm ill it's all fallen on her.
Doctor:	How long have you and Judy been married?
Jack:	It's our silver wedding next year.
Doctor:	And children?
Jack:	A son. He is one of these computer whiz kids. Salary nearly as good as mine was, and still only 23!

In this sequence Jack does not feel that anything he has said is unacceptable; but he has been neatly steered away from expressing his feelings to talking about his family in general terms. His concerns about his relationship with Judy remain unaddressed; yet the focus has been switched in such a way that the doctor is not perceived as uninterested. However, had the doctor explored Jack's concerns, he would have been perceived as *more* interested in Jack as a person.

Neutral material is often used to change topic or focus. Sometimes this material is offered by the patient; but more commonly it is introduced by the health professional, and often justified on the grounds of 'wishing to take his mind off morbid thoughts'. This type of distancing works because it controls the subjects of the patients' interactions and maintains the exchange at a relatively superficial level.

Some patients, however, perhaps because they are assertive, or because the extent of their worry is so great, refuse to be controlled in this way. One of the distancing tactics used with such patients is called 'passing the buck'.

Passing the buck

If questions and concerns continue to be raised, in spite of health professionals' attempts to distance, it is often convenient to 'pass the buck' to colleagues, on the grounds that they will be more informed and better able to deal with the matter. This distancing technique is quite different from genuine referral, where the person being asked the question does *not* have enough information to answer.

The nurse with the menus, for example, knew that Fred's disease had progressed to a level which was inoperable; but she did not wish to be the person to break the bad news and deal with the consequent emotional reactions. The next time she was by his bed, Fred again tried to gain information, and by now was feeling frustrated and irritated:

Fred:	Can you spare a minute, nurse?
Nurse:	Yes, Fred, have you settled in?
Fred:	No, and I won't until someone tells me what is going on.
Nurse:	[looking puzzled] But I thought they had.
Fred:	[getting angry] You know what I mean ... 'a few cancerous cells—more tests—rest'. My cousin had an operation and then died in three years—and where does that leave me? Too far gone to operate?
Nurse:	Please, Fred, don't get angry with me. The doctors should have answered your questions.
Fred:	But why can't you—you must know what is going on!
Nurse:	This is something for the doctor. I'm sure he will talk to you if you ask.

The nurse made her escape as soon as possible, leaving Fred both angry and convinced that things were worse than he had expected. Of course, many nurses would argue that they are not allowed to give information to patients. This is not usually the case, and is in fact a different issue—one which is addressed later in this book.

All health professionals may use passing the buck as a distancing tactic. This not only includes the plea that they are not the person to ask, but also laying blame when things go wrong, or deferring decision-making. Far from giving comfort, such strategies can result in considerable stress and anxiety for the patient.

Premature problem-solving

Sometimes, there is an attempt to solve the patient's (or relatives') problems before exploring the nature of the problem or its relationship to other facets of the individual's life. Again this allows the professional to be seen to fulfil his/her role while maintaining interaction at a superficial level.

Jill Hilton had difficulties with her partner and their sexual relationship. She was worried that this would cause problems when she went home. She tried to share her worries with the doctor:

Jill:	I'm worried about going home.
Doctor:	Don't be worried, I'm sure your family will be supportive. I'm sure your partner understands.

Jill: That's just it.
Doctor: Is it the sexual side of things? Well, you will know
                when it feels right. He knows he must be patient. I'm
                sure you can think of ways to let him know you are
                ready—candlelight dinner, soft music, ha ha.
Jill: But ...
Doctor: Now don't worry—I know your family are delighted
                that you are going home.

When Jill said 'but' she wanted to explain that her husband was in fact
'turned off' if ever she made the first approach, and that her problems
were at a very different level. If the doctor had explored her concerns
he would have discovered that she believed that she had 'caught cancer'
from her husband. She had read that promiscuity causes cervical cancer
due to dirty foreskins, and had concluded that, since she was not
promiscuous, her husband must carry the 'germ' in his penis.

From the above it can be seen that premature problem-solving can
leave patients tense and frustrated, with the belief that no one has time
to understand their real problems. If Jill survives mentally, she may one
day laugh at the idea of trying to take the lead with a man who has to be
totally in control in the sexual arena.

Another danger with premature problem-solving is that, because the
interaction has stayed at a superficial level, the real problems do not
emerge. With Jill the doctor made a correct educated guess that Jill's
distress was sexual, but did not focus on the nature of the problem. All
health professionals are not so lucky, and may spend considerable time
in offering solutions to problems that are on the periphery of the main
concern, which, were it known, would make the solutions offered appear
totally inappropriate.

Avoiding the patient
The ultimate distancing strategy is physically to avoid the patient who
has obvious fears and worries. Rather like the waiter who will not catch
your eye in a restaurant, the nurse or doctor hurries by the bed,
seemingly unaware of the patient's attempt to gain someone's attention.
Junior staff are sent to care for the patient physically, and doctors say a
cheery 'Good morning' at the foot of the bed and move on rapidly.

This strategy can have far-reaching effects for the professional and
the patient. Stockwell (1972) found that once a patient is avoided by one
member of staff, he or she is soon labelled by all staff, and becomes
'the unpopular patient'. Stockwell found that this could happen to any

patient who did not conform to the expectations of the staff, who wish their patients to be cheerful, helpful, and determined to get better quickly. It can be seen that the patient who is worried and anxious, asks difficult questions, and comes to negative conclusions about his or her prognosis, is high on the list for being avoided and unpopular.

The patients, with time on their hands, try to make sense of the situation, and may become withdrawn and introspective, if not frustrated and angry. They then fall into the added role of the difficult patient, whom nurses may describe as withdrawn. In other words the patients are seen as the ones who are distancing.

Patient distancing
There are many reasons put forward to explain the fact that patients do not always seem prepared to share their concerns with health professionals. It is hypothesized that uniform may be a barrier, that patients perceive the staff to be 'too busy', and that they feel that their concerns are trivial compared with those of 'really ill' people, and that they should be grateful for receiving care and treatment.

It is a fact that any individuals who find themselves in a strange environment, having to deal with new experiences, will call on past experience to make sense of the current dilemma. It is reasonable to suggest that most patients will have only a social or work experience to call on. In a new social situation, most people sum up the situation and make a decision (albeit unconsciously) to conform or to remain very individual and take the consequences. In a new job there is more pressure to conform, as there is in circumstances which are frightening.

It is suggested here that most patients take their lead from the health professionals and other conforming patients. In most of the distancing strategies used by health professionals there is a social norm to reinforce the strategy. Uniform may be added to the list of barriers created, but is far less potent than the strategies themselves.

There is some debate as to whether distancing strategies are con-sciously used to block the patients. Certainly they can be habitual, having been found to be an effective mechanism to protect the pro-fessional from the true emotional cost of care. It will also be seen, in Chapter 1, that there are specific, well-documented reasons why patients with cancer use distancing tactics.

In the following chapters we will propose a model of care which is based on the identification of patients' concerns from the individual's perspective. That there is a cost is accepted, and this will be addressed;

but health professionals using the model report enhanced job satisfaction.

Summary

In this chapter the reasons why health professionals distance themselves from their patients have been considered. Many strategies have been described, including the use of neutral material, ignoring or selectively attending to cues, the use of inappropriate encouragement or reassurance, switching the topic, premature problem-solving, and active avoidance of the patient. It has been suggested that such strategies are used in the belief that it is a kindness to soften the patient's reality.

References

Faulkner, A. and Maguire, P. (1984). Teaching assessment skills. In *Recent Advances in Nursing 7: Communication* (ed. A. Faulkner), pp. 130–45. Churchill Livingstone, Edinburgh.

Stockwell, F. (1972). *The unpopular patient*. Royal College of Nursing, London.

3

Patient assessment: structure and content

Introduction

The aim of an initial assessment is to establish which problems concern the patient, whether they be physical, social, psychological, or spiritual. The health professional should interview in a way which engenders trust and promotes compliance with advice and treatment. Beginning the interview; assessing the current problems and their impact; and ending the interview form three distinct parts of the assessment.

Beginning the interview

Before assessing someone, it is important for the health professional to decide on the strategy to be used. When time is short or the referral letter mentions an overriding problem, it is important to focus on the present situation. Otherwise, the health professional should invite the patient to give a history of the onset and development of his or her problems from their beginning to the present time. This allows insight into patients' experience of disease and treatment, together with their perceptions of these and their impact on their daily lives, moods, and personal relationships. This scene-setting strategy is important in that it encourages patients to articulate problems, and then they can be invited to put them in priority order, and to focus on the main one if time is short.

If the health professional is seeing a newly referred patient there is a danger that he or she might be biased by the content of the referral letter and miss other important concerns that the patient has not mentioned. It is important to check patients' beliefs on those concerns most pertinent to them.

Setting

Whenever possible, the patient should be seen in private and alone. If this is not possible, an illusion of privacy should be given by drawing screens or by sitting apart from others in the room. Otherwise, disclosure of important information may be inhibited because of embarrassment or fears about upsetting relatives, close friends, or other patients. If a friend or relative wishes to be present, it may be necessary to point out the importance of talking to the patient alone and to offer to see the relative later. In the home setting, it may be necessary to be very firm.

Mr Hancock:	Hello. Who are you?
Nurse Smithers:	I'm the Macmillan nurse. Dr Blow asked me to come round to see if I could help your wife in any way.
Mr Hancock:	Do come in. She is through there, in the sitting-room.
Nurse Smithers:	It would be helpful if I could see her on my own at first and then I could talk to you later.
Mr Hancock:	I will come with you.
Nurse Smithers:	I do find it is much better if I can talk to each person separately, and so I would very much like to talk to her first and then talk to you afterwards.
Mr Hancock:	I suppose that's all right. I'd better take you through.

Orientating the patient

If the assessment visit represents the first time the patient has seen the health professional, his or her expectations of how you are going to behave will be based on his or her earlier experience of health professionals. Negotiation on what you plan to do should overcome anxieties of this nature. A first step is to introduce and explain who you are working with, why you are there, and the time you plan to spend with the patient, and to mention that you would like to take notes. Such an introduction might go as follows:

Dr Johnston:	Hello, I'm Dr Johnston. I work with Professor Smith in the Oncology Department. What I would like to do today is to talk with you to establish just what your main problems are and then discuss what we might be able to do about them. I have up to 20 minutes if we need it, and I would like to take some notes to help remind me of what we have discussed. Is that all right?
Mr Seymour:	Yes, that's fine.

Explaining the time available

Many health professionals fear that telling patients how much time is available will put them off and make them feel that they are not cared for. However, offering 15 minutes or more leaves most patients feeling that they do not have enough of interest to tell the health professional in the available time. Being explicit with patients about the time available encourages them to pace themselves, so that they disclose their main concerns rather than talking about unimportant matters.

When the amount of time available is mentioned some patients may object that it is insufficient. You should then indicate that you will get as far as you can in the time you have available, but will see the patient again soon to clarify any outstanding matters. Once you have negotiated time in this way it is very important not to be drawn into a much longer interview than you have agreed. By avoiding 'neutral' material, such as questions about the patient's mode of travel to the clinic or hospital, it will be clear that the interview is about the patient's concerns, and will follow the pattern and time-limits agreed.

Dr Johnston: What I would like to do, but only if you agree, is to take you back to the beginning when you first became ill. Is that all right?

Mr Seymour: Yes.

Dr Johnston: OK. What was the first thing you noticed that went wrong?

Mr Seymour: I started coughing up blood.

Note-taking

Many health professionals worry that taking notes will suggest to patients that you are not interested in what they are saying. On the contrary, note-taking, particularly if it records key utterances, will be seen by the patient as evidence that you are listening properly. Moreover, it is not possible to remember all the cues given by a patient unless you take systematic notes. These need not be lengthy, but should include key words and phrases. Looking up at patients at the end of each key utterance will indicate that you are really interested in what they are saying.

The professional's versus the patient's agenda

Traditionally, the health professional asks a series of questions in a predetermined sequence in order to cover key areas that will allow a diagnosis or an assessment of current problems to be made. However, interviewing is more effective if the health professional first focuses on the patient's agenda (Stewart *et al.* 1986)—that is, on the areas the patient perceives to be important—before covering any remaining areas that have not been volunteered.

Health professionals may fear that a patient-led agenda will waste time. In practice, it saves time, because the important facts are disclosed earlier in the interview, and there is often much less need to ask routine check questions, such as 'Have you had any problems with your breathing?', because the answer to this will already have emerged as part of the patient's account of his or her illness. Contrast the following interactions:

Example 1

Dr Smith:	Can you tell me what has been the problem?
Mrs Poole:	I found a breast lump.
Dr Smith:	When did you notice that?
Mrs Poole:	Six weeks ago.
Dr Smith:	Where was it?
Mrs Poole:	In my left breast.
Dr Smith:	Has it been painful?
Mrs Poole:	No.
Dr Smith:	Did it change in any way when you had your period?
Mrs Poole:	No.
Dr Smith:	Has it changed in size since you found it?
Mrs Poole:	No.
Dr Smith:	Has there been any discharge from your nipple?
Mrs Poole:	No.
Dr Smith:	Have you noticed any changes in your skin?
Mrs Poole:	No.
Dr Smith:	Have you ever had breast lumps before?
Mrs Poole:	No.

Example 2

Dr Smith:	What have been the problems that have brought you here today?
Mrs Poole:	I found a lump in my left breast.
Dr Smith:	When was that?
Mrs Poole:	Six weeks ago.
Dr Smith:	Can you tell me how you felt about finding the lump?
Mrs Poole:	I thought, 'What next!' My father had died a month before—so of course I thought the worst.
Dr Smith:	The worst?
Mrs Poole:	Well, dad died of cancer, you see—and it all seems to be coming at once. Ted—my husband—he's just been made redundant.

Dr Smith:	So, you have had a whole pile of problems on your plate?
Mrs Poole:	Yes.
Dr Smith:	Do you mind if I just check if there are any other problems before we go into the ones you have mentioned?
Mrs Poole:	No, though I keep worrying that other things will go wrong.
Dr Smith:	It must be difficult for you—but I wonder which of these problems would you like me to focus on first.
Mrs Poole:	My lump—I'm so scared it could be cancer.

In Example 1, the doctor is asking a series of important questions in relation to the nature of a patient's breast lump in order to determine whether it is likely to be benign or cancerous. Clearly, such questions are important; but this is a very limited form of interviewing. It results in the patient often responding merely with a 'No.' Contrast this with the patient-led approach. Instead of assuming that Mrs Poole wants help with her breast problem first, the doctor negotiated with Mrs Poole by asking 'Which of these problems would you like me to focus on first?' She did in fact give priority to her breast lump, but had been given the opportunity to focus on other concerns, before Dr Smith moved on to the nature and extent of the primary problem.

As the doctor proceeds, he or she should stay with a patient-led agenda, and attempt to elicit the information spontaneously from the patient before asking any directive questions. For example, when Mrs Poole is questioned about her father's death the dialogue goes as follows:

Dr Smith:	I can see how worried you are about your breast lump, but I wonder if you want to talk about your other problems?
Mrs Poole:	Well, losing dad has been terrible.
Dr Smith:	Can you tell me about that?
Mrs Poole:	He had cancer—he went down so fast.
Dr Smith:	How has that affected you?
Mrs Poole:	I have become ever so depressed.
Dr Smith:	Depressed? Could you tell me exactly what you have noticed?
Mrs Poole:	I have just got so low I feel in a black pit; I can't get out of it. I can't sleep, I keep waking through the night, I have just lost interest in things. I have no energy. I cry all the time. I have felt ever so irritable.

	I have so little energy, and everything is an increasing effort. I find myself preoccupied with thoughts of him all the time.
Dr Smith:	Have you noticed any other changes?
Mrs Poole:	I can't concentrate: I can't be bothered to watch the television or read. In fact I don't know what to do with myself.
Dr Smith:	Any other changes during this time?
Mrs Poole:	No, except for this lump [starts to cry].

Mrs Poole has already volunteered most of the symptoms of depression. Not all patients will be so articulate as Mrs Poole, nor will they necessarily cover all areas of concern to the doctor. This may mean that, although the agenda is primarily patient-led, elements of a professional agenda will also crop up, either within the interview in response to cues, or at the end to cover areas that have been omitted in the patient's account of the situation. Dr Smith, for example, will move into a professional agenda to elicit whether Mrs Poole has other symptoms of depression, including thoughts of suicide.

Areas to be covered
Given that a patient-led agenda does not follow a pre-set pattern, it is important that the following areas are covered.

1. *History of the patient's illness*
It is important to elicit the history of the patient's illness from the time of onset of the first symptoms, in order to determine exactly how it presented and how the patient responded, as in the following example:

Dr Pearce:	When did you first notice the lump?
Mrs Banks:	Six weeks ago, just after the August Bank holiday.
Dr Pearce:	What exactly did you notice?
Mrs Banks:	A small hard lump.
Dr Pearce:	Where exactly was it?
Mrs Banks:	It was in my left breast. I tried to ignore it; I hoped it would go away, but it didn't. That's why I'm here now.
Dr Pearce:	How have you been feeling about it?
Mrs Banks:	Very worried. I thought it might be cancer, because at my age, well, there is a strong possibility.
Dr Pearce:	Any other reasons you are worrying it might be cancer?

Mrs Banks:	No, I just know it is a strong possibility.
Dr Pearce:	Well, can I ask you a few more questions about the nature of your lump? And then I'll examine you and see if your fears are justified.

Here the practitioner has established the history of the key symptoms and also checked the patient's awareness of what the diagnosis might be and her response to it.

2. *Seeking advice*

It is important to discover when the patient first sought medical advice, what happened, and how the patient perceived the information and advice given. In particular, it is important to determine whether help was prompt and relevant or whether there was undue delay and inappropriate advice. If there were problems with the initial handling of the patient's complaints, what were the patient's reactions? Distrust may have developed towards all health professionals, and this may have hindered the patient's psychological adaptation to his or her predicament. Mr Renton was referred to a medical oncologist:

Dr Carruthers:	You say you went to your general practitioner immediately you noticed that the mole was getting bigger?
Mr Renton:	Yes. He warned me it could be a kind of cancer, and that we shouldn't mess about with it. So the mole was excised and biopsied a few days later.
Dr Carruthers:	And how did that turn out?
Mr Renton:	It turned out to be a melanoma; but they said they had caught it early. They advised me to see you because you are an expert on melanoma and have some drugs that should make all the cancer go.
Dr Carruthers:	How have you been feeling about all this?
Mr Renton:	I was shattered by the idea of having cancer; but I am relieved that you might have some treatment that will get rid of it.

While Mr Renton was clearly aware of his diagnosis, the situation may not be so straightforward for other patients:

Dr Smith:	Can I go back to when you first found your lump and saw your GP?
Mrs Vincent:	Yes.
Dr Smith:	What happened?

Mrs Vincent:	He examined me, and said it was nothing to worry about. It was a lump that would go away. He advised me to come back if it didn't. I left it a good two months before I went back; but the lump was still there. I also noticed the puckering of my skin.
Dr Smith:	And then?
Mrs Vincent:	He sent me to a surgeon, who didn't see me for three weeks because my appointment got lost in the post. He eventually found out it was cancer. Since then I can't help feeling that the whole thing would have been different if people had acted sooner. As it is I am told my chances are not very good.
Dr Smith:	How do you mean?
Mrs Vincent:	Well, they say it is only 50–50.

3. Impact of treatment

It is important to elicit how patients perceive the treatment they are receiving and the extent to which their daily lives have been affected in several key areas of functioning. Useful questions include: 'What treatments have you been having so far?'; and 'How has the treatment been affecting you?' In exploring this it is important to name each specific treatment, such as chemotherapy or radiotherapy, in turn. It is then useful to ask 'What has the impact been on your day-to-day life?'; 'What about your ability to do your chores?'; and 'Has it had any affect on your ability to continue working, and to maintain your normal social life, hobbies, and interests?' It is particularly important to ask if there has been any effect on the patient's relationship with his or her partner and what the effects may have been on their sexual relationship. It is also important to elicit the effect on the patient's ability to concentrate, and on his or her mood. Such questions should prompt honest disclosure of adverse effects which would otherwise have remained hidden. For example, this patient was very concerned about the side-effects of treatment:

Nurse Jones:	You say you have been having chemotherapy to get rid of this lung trouble. How has it been affecting you?
Ms Parr:	Not too bad.
Nurse Jones:	What do you mean, 'Not too bad'?
Ms Parr:	Well, I have had some sickness.
Nurse Jones:	Some sickness?
Ms Parr:	Yes; at times it has been pretty bad.

Nurse Jones:	Pretty bad?
Ms Parr:	Well, to be honest it has been so bad I have thought of giving it up. I just can't bear the thought of any more.
Nurse Jones:	Can you bear to tell me just how bad it has been?
Ms Parr:	At times I can't stop being sick, particularly after the infusion.
Nurse Jones:	But just how sick have you been?
Ms Parr:	I vomit non-stop for the whole day after the injection.
Nurse Jones:	Have you told anybody about it before today?

4. The current status of the patient's disease and its impact
It is necessary to check with patients how things appear at the present time from their perspective.

Dr Brown:	What is the state of play now, Mr Grimes?
Mr Grimes:	The hospital have told me it is all clear.
Dr Brown:	How do you feel about that?
Mr Grimes:	Very pleased. It is what I hoped for. When I heard it was the Big C I thought I was done for.
Dr Brown:	So, are you saying now that everything is fine?
Mr Grimes:	Yes, there are no problems. I feel fine.

With a different patient the result of this enquiry revealed that there were serious problems:

Dr Foster:	How have you been since I saw you last?
Mr Brownlow:	Very poorly. My breathlessness is worse. I can hardly walk upstairs. I guess that's because my cancer is now spreading.
Dr Foster:	It looks like it. But I need to examine you and do some more X-rays to check this out. Even so, we should be able to help you with these symptoms.
Mr Brownlow:	I hope so, because really I am not sure that the quality of my life is worth it at the moment.
Dr Foster:	That sounds very grim for you.
Mr Brownlow:	It is.
Dr Foster:	Are you experiencing any other physical problems apart from your breathlessness?
Mr Brownlow:	Isn't that enough?
Dr Foster:	I'm sorry; but it is important that I check what problems you are having, even though I know it is tough for you.

5. *Current psychological state*

You should establish how the patient has been coping, and whether there is any evidence of psychological or psychiatric morbidity. A useful way to do this is to check how the patient is coping with his or her adaptation to the diagnosis of cancer (see Chapter 1) and any treatment.

6. *Current mood state*

It is critical to assess a patient's mood state, particularly as anxiety and depression can cause great mental suffering and lower the threshold at which physical symptoms such as pain are experienced. Consequently, if these psychological states are present the physical suffering will be intensified. If the patient does not offer cues, questions should be asked, such as 'Have you felt particularly low, miserable, or depressed at any stage since you became ill?' (to elicit depressed mood); or 'Have you felt particularly tense, on edge, or unable to relax since you became ill?' (to elicit anxious mood). If the patient answers 'yes' you should check whether the changed mood represents a distinct departure from the patient's normal mood, and has been accompanied by four or more of the established symptoms of anxiety or depression (Chapter 1).

If depression is present it is vital to check whether there is any risk of suicide by asking explicit questions about it.

Suicidal risk

Health professionals often fear that exploring suicidal risk will create conflict, because the patient will object strongly to being asked the relevant questions. There may also be conflict because patients believe they have a right to suicide and that the health professional has no excuse for trying to interfere. It is important to know how to explore suicidal risk and to make appropriate judgements about management. When any patient presents with symptoms of depression, questions about suicidal risk are mandatory, including questions about the patients' perceptions of the future. It is also important to screen for hopelessness and guilt, and for contrast with previous thoughts and feelings.

Dr Matthews:	You say you have felt low for some months. Just what are you like at your lowest?
Mr Owen:	I just see no point in going on.
Dr Matthews:	You say you see no point in going on; have you ever felt so low you have felt like ending your life?
Mr Owen:	Yes. I have.

Dr Matthews:	What exactly have you considered?
Mr Owen:	I thought of electrocuting myself in the bath.
Dr Matthews:	How close have you come to doing that?
Mr Owen:	Well, it's occurred to me on at least three occasions that it is something I should do to end all this misery; but I haven't quite been able to bring myself to do it, though I am frightened I could.
Dr Matthews:	What has held you back?
Mr Owen:	The thought of what it would do to my wife and children. That's the only thing that has held me back. But now it's getting harder and harder to resist.
Dr Matthews:	How are you feeling about yourself as a person at the moment?
Mr Owen:	I feel I am no use to anyone; I just feel a burden. As my disease gets worse and I get weaker, I think I am becoming far too much for the family, particularly Barbara, to handle. I think they would be better off without me. I feel so guilty and hopeless—not like myself at all.

By the end of this, Dr Matthews had identified suicidal plans and that the patient was about to act on them. While the conversation also revealed important protective factors, notably concern about his wife and children, these were no longer sufficient to prevent him trying to kill himself. The interview also revealed ideas of pointlessness, feelings of there being no future, and feelings of guilt, of unworthiness, and of being a burden. All these carry a high risk of suicide; so it was appropriate that Dr Matthews firmly confronted Mr Owen with the need for treatment:

Mr Owen:	It's my life—I'm at the end of my tether.
Dr Matthews:	Mr Owen, you need help right now with your underlying depression. It is that which is making you feel suicidal.
Mr Owen:	But anyone in my position would want to end it.
Dr Matthews:	I can understand how you feel; but you have a depressive but treatable illness, and we can help you with that.

Other features of suicidal risk worth exploring include increasing age, a past history of suicide attempts, recent loss (such as a bereavement or redundancy), being socially isolated, and experiencing chronic problems such as housing or financial difficulties.

When patients cannot give you an undertaking not to kill themselves, this represents an emergency. An immediate expert psychiatric assessment is warranted; but someone must stay with the patient until a medical opinion is obtained.

7. Overall level of functioning
It is important to establish whether the illness and treatment have had any adverse effects on the patient's ability to work and cope with household chores, social and leisure activities, and key personal relationships. If adverse effects are present it is important to clarify the exact nature and causes of the problems.

Dr Raeburn:	You say you have been getting out much less since you started radiotherapy. Why is that?
Mrs Cross:	I feel so unclean.
Dr Raeburn:	Would you like to tell me more about that?
Mrs Cross:	Well, as you know, I have had cancer of the cervix, and had both surgery and radiotherapy. I have felt increasingly dirty because everybody says you only get this cancer because you have been promiscuous. I have been terrified that people must think I'm a prostitute. I have become more and more self-conscious about it, and got to the stage of thinking it would be better not to go out at all. It is a stigma. I don't feel I can fight it.
Dr Raeburn:	Have there been any other changes in you as a result of the treatment?
Mrs Cross:	I can't stand love-making any more. But I don't know how my husband is putting up with this at the moment. I have not been able to return to work because I am worried about what the other women are thinking. I have really become a recluse. I only feel safe in the house.

8. Level of disclosure
When systematic enquiry reveals that problems are evident it is important to check whether they have been disclosed to anybody in a position to help, and to elicit the impact on key relationships:

Dr Raeburn:	Have you been able to tell your husband how you have felt about love-making?

Mrs Cross:	No. I just made excuses that I was sore. But I think he knows it is more than that.
Dr Raeburn:	How has he been responding?
Mrs Cross:	He was very tolerant at first, but he has got increasingly irritable in recent weeks. He says he can't understand it, because he tells me how much he loves me but I don't want to know.
Dr Raeburn:	And how are things at the moment?
Mrs Cross:	I think he is bewildered; but I can't tell him the truth.
Dr Raeburn:	How has all this affected your relationship with your husband?
Mrs Cross:	We are arguing a lot more. He seems to be running out of patience with me. He thinks I should be back to work already.

Sometimes the patient has attempted to disclose problems, but had a negative response from her partner:

Nurse Spinks:	You say that you tried to tell your husband that you were feeling upset about your stoma. How did he take it?
Mrs Blow:	He said he just didn't want to talk about it. He said he has enough on his plate with all the problems at work, and it was only going to upset him if we did talk about it.
Nurse Spinks:	And how are you feeling about that at the moment?
Mrs Blow:	I feel rejected. I felt he wasn't interested in what had happened to me. I have begun to wonder if there is much future in our relationship.
Nurse Spinks:	Has he always found things like this distressing?
Mrs Blow:	Yes. He has never liked talking to me about feelings. He copes by 'sweeping things under the carpet'. But it hurts me so much. I really begin to think he doesn't care.

9. *Other important life events*

There may have been other adverse events in the patient's or relative's recent past that may have contributed to their current predicament. Such difficulties may include recent bereavement, financial difficulties, or unemployment. Questions should be asked to allow disclosure of these problems, and to identify their exact nature and extent, if they have been disclosed, the level of response, and how the patient is feeling about his or her future.

Ending the interview

When all key areas have been covered as part of the patient's agenda, or by the health professional, a clear picture should emerge of the patient's current problems. It is then useful to leave enough time to recap what you have learned and check with the patient that what you have heard is correct. Only when the current problems have been fully established and clarified should any attempt be made to discuss with the patient what problems they would most like help with and to discuss the need for further investigation or ways of resolving the problems.

Summary

It is important to have a clear beginning, middle, and end to the assessment interview, and to be aware of the areas to be covered. Ideally, these should be cued by the patient and followed up accordingly. Once the patient's disclosures have been exhausted it may then be necessary for the health professional to ask a series of questions to determine the exact nature, duration, and intensity of a given problem. It is important to try to ensure that a full problem list has been established before beginning to discuss with the patient what information is needed about the nature of the problem and its investigation and treatment.

References

Stewart, M. A., Brown, J. B., Levenstein, J. H., McCracken, E., and McWhinney, I. R. (1986). The patient-centred clinical method. 3. Changes in resident's performance over 2 months of training. *Family Practice—An International Journal*, **3**, 164–7.

4

Patient assessment: skills

Initial assessment
If health professionals are to establish the exact nature and extent of their patients' main problems, they need to develop skills that promote disclosure, and avoid using those that make people less likely to disclose their concerns.

Behaviour that can inhibit disclosure
Before beginning an assessment interview it is important that the interviewer is aware that certain behaviours inhibit the patient from disclosing key problems and that the use of these is avoided whenever possible. These behaviours include the use of closed questions, for example, 'Have you had any difficulty with breathing lately?' This invites a yes or no answer, and doesn't encourage patients to volunteer any more information about their experience of particular symptoms. The more closed questions that are asked, the lower the level of disclosure.

When the patient is presenting with a predominantly physical problem it is inevitable that the interviewer will want to spend time focusing on and clarifying the nature of the physical symptoms before raising any social, psychological, or spiritual issues. However, it has been established that the longer the time the interviewer focuses on physical aspects, the more likely the patient is to believe that the interviewer is not interested in other problems. This 'programming' can happen early on in an interview, and can seriously hinder the disclosure of social, psychological, or spiritual problems.

The problem for the health professional is how to integrate physical, social, and psychological enquiry early on in an interview without impeding the important function of identifying the nature of the illness.

For example, the following brief history was taken from a woman who presented with a breast lump:

Mr Farrell: As you know, your GP referred you to me because you have a breast lump. When did you first notice it?
Mrs Broadhurst: Six weeks ago.
Mr Farrell: What did it feel like?
Mrs Broadhurst: It felt hard, like a marble in my left breast.
Mr Farrell: Did it change at all in relation to your period?
Mrs Broadhurst: No.
Mr Farrell: Have you ever had this kind of lump before?
Mrs Broadhurst: No.
Mr Farrell: Has there been any discharge from your nipple?
Mrs Broadhurst: No.
Mr Farrell: Has it been painful at all?
Mrs Broadhurst: No.

In the above exchange, closed questions elicited the facts of Mrs Broadhurst's physical condition but did not include her feelings or perceptions of the current situation. Compare that with the following exchange:

Mr Farrell: When did you notice this lump?
Mrs Broadhurst: Six weeks ago. I was having a bath and I checked myself as usual. I felt this lump in my left breast.
Mr Farrell: What was it like?
Mrs Broadhurst: It was hard, like a marble.
Mr Farrell: What did you think it might be?
Mrs Broadhurst: I immediately thought I had breast cancer.
Mr Farrell: How did that make you feel?
Mrs Broadhurst: Extremely worried. In fact I have not been able to stop worrying since, because my mother had breast cancer and died of it after only two years. I have been terrified about what you would say to me about it today.
Mr Farrell: Can I just check if there have been any other changes?
Mrs Broadhurst: I don't think there have.
Mr Farrell: For example, has your lump changed in size in relation to your period?
Mrs Broadhurst: No.
Mr Farrell: Has there been any discharge from your nipple?
Mrs Broadhurst: No.

In the latter example, the surgeon has indicated early on that he is genuinely interested in knowing how Mrs Broadhurst had perceived her lump and reacted to it. This interview has taken a little more time, but Mrs Broadhurst is now more likely to disclose her concerns rather than to focus purely on the physical aspects of her disease.

When patients disclose problems—for example, when Mrs Broadhurst says she felt terrified because she thought she had cancer like her mother, and implies that she believes she might also die from her disease in two years—it can be very tempting for the surgeon to move immediately into reassurance or advice mode. Thus, Mr Farrell might say, 'Oh, I'm sure your illness isn't as serious as your mother's', or 'Despite what happened to your mother, our treatments are so much better these days; so let me tell you what we can do about it.'

Faced with premature and inappropriate advice and reassurance, the patient will still be worried, but will feel that she cannot disclose her concerns. However, worry about these concerns will prevent her heeding the advice given. Hence it is important to elicit all concerns and to establish their nature and intensity *before* giving any advice or reassurance.

Leading questions, where the question implies the desired answer, also inhibit disclosure. For example, 'Things are going well, aren't they?' presupposes agreement, whereas in fact the patient may be very concerned about the way things are going.

Similarly, multiple questions, where several questions are asked at the same time, can inhibit disclosure, because the patient will normally respond to only one of the questions. The others may then be 'lost', even though they are an important element of the overall assessment:

Dr Jones: You say you have been having problems with your arm since surgery. Have you been having any pain? How well can you move your arm? How much does it interfere with your daily life?

Mrs Bond: The pain is terrific, it really is keeping me awake at night.

Dr Jones then concentrated on the patient's pain, and did not return to the other issues.

Skills that can promote disclosure
In order to establish the full nature and extent of a patient's problems, key skills are required. Table 4.1 lists these skills, and the corresponding poor techniques that may inhibit disclosure.

Table 4.1 Effect of interviewing skills on patient disclosure

Promoting	Inhibiting
Questions:	Questions:
open-directive	closed
psychological focus	multiple
screening	leading
Precision	Clarification—
Prompting	physical focus
Cue-responding	Advice
Clarifying psychological aspects	Reassurance
Control	Premature advice
Empathy	Premature reassurance
Educated guesses	

Precision

It is important that you encourage patients to make an effort to be exact about when particular events occurred. This will enable them to remember exactly what happened, to connect with the associated emotions, and to describe both their experiences and their feelings about them more accurately.

Dr Johnston: When exactly did you begin to notice you were coughing up blood?

Mr Seymour: Oh, towards the end of last year.

Dr Johnston: Exactly when? Can you try and remember? It would be helpful.

Mr Seymour: It was early in December, my daughter had just had her birthday.

Open directive questions

Since patients may be genuinely reluctant to disclose their perceptions and feelings, or any social or psychological problems, it is useful not only to be precise, but early on in the interview to ask questions that unambiguously convey that you have a real interest in understanding how the patient has been feeling. A typical interview might proceed as follows:

Dr Johnston: When you noticed you were coughing up blood, did *you* have any idea what it might be due to?
Mr Seymour: I was worried it might be cancer.
Dr Johnston: Why did you think that?
Mr Seymour: I'm a heavy smoker, and I know that one of the first signs of lung cancer can be coughing up blood.
Dr Johnston: So, how did that leave you feeling?
Mr Seymour: Terrified that it could be cancer. It might mean the end of my life.

Such open directive questions (in this case questions about what the bleeding might be due to, and about how it left the patient feeling) encourage patients to elaborate on their experiences in relation to the focus of the question, rather than just giving yes or no answers.

Prompting

When the scene-setting strategy has been negotiated with a patient and accepted, it is important to help patients to stay in chronological sequence, in order to increase the likelihood that they will give accurate and relevant histories. This can best be achieved by repeatedly prompting the patient—by saying, for example, 'Right', 'Yes', 'Go on', or 'What happened next?' This encourages patients to complete one sequence at a time without wandering from the point. Otherwise patients tend to introduce other problems before they have fully elaborated the first one. It is here that the techniques of control are important.

Control

Here the interviewer is seeking to get the patient back into sequence or to talking about a particular problem that he or she hadn't fully elaborated. It is important that this is done the moment the interviewer senses that the sequence is being lost or that he or she is being side-tracked on to another problem. Without this level of control it is easy to forget what has happened, and to fail to return to the original issues. Important information is then missing at the end of the assessment. In seeking to control the interview in this sense it is important to establish with the patient that this is being done in order to get back to the sequence or to a particular problem, rather than to avoid the additional problems that are now being introduced, and to negotiate the acceptability of this:

Dr Johnston: Apart from coughing up blood in early December, did you notice any other changes?

Mr Seymour: I was beginning to go off my food and to lose weight. I was also having trouble with my right knee. It kept locking, and was very painful at times. It was extremely frustrating, and I had physiotherapy for it. But it wasn't getting any better.

Dr Johnston: Yes, I can understand that your knee has been a problem for you; but can I just take you back to the problems relating to your coughing up blood. We can talk about your knee problem later.

Mr Seymour: Yes, OK.

In focusing on the patient's agenda Dr Johnston avoided making assumptions about the presenting complaint. He has found out about three key problems (haemoptysis, and loss of appetite and weight).

Summarizing

It is helpful if Dr Johnston summarizes what he has understood from the patient before screening for any other concerns. This gives Mr Seymour a chance to correct him if he has misunderstood the nature of these concerns; and it also indicates to the patient that his concerns have been heard and registered.

Dr Johnston: So far you have mentioned that you started coughing up blood early in December last year, and noticed a loss of appetite and weight. You also mentioned that you were very worried it might be cancer. I would like to go into those concerns a little more.

Mr Seymour: Right.

Screening questions

It would be tempting for Dr Johnston to believe that he has elicited all Mr Seymour's key problems. However, it is important that he should screen for the possibility that there may be other problems, as yet undisclosed, which may be even more important than those so far revealed. He can best do this by asking a screening question:

Dr Johnston: You mentioned that you have been coughing up blood, you have lost your appetite and are losing weight, and

you are very worried it might be cancer. I would like
to talk to you about these problems in more detail; but
before I do so, could you tell me if you have any other
problems?

Mr Seymour: No, everything else seems quite normal.

Dr Johnston can now be reasonably confident that no problems are being
withheld from him, and can concentrate on clarifying those elicited
already.

Clarification

In clarifying concerns Dr Johnston is seeking to understand their exact
nature, intensity, and duration. He is particularly trying to understand
what it was like from the patient's viewpoint. He is also seeking to create
a climate where as the patient clarifies the nature of his experiences he
feels more able to disclose and express any associated feelings, rather
than just presenting his concerns or problems in a neutral manner:

Dr Johnston: Can I start then with your coughing up blood. What
exactly was happening?

Mr Seymour: I thought it was just my usual smoker's cough, but I
found myself coughing a lot.

Dr Johnston: When you say 'a lot', just how often were you
coughing?

Mr Seymour: Initially I suppose five, six times a day, and maybe
bringing up blood once or twice; but then early in the
new year I was coughing several times every hour,
and bringing up blood several times a day.

Dr Johnston: Were you bringing up any phlegm?

Mr Seymour: No, just blood.

Dr Johnston: You said you were losing weight at the time: just how
much weight had you lost by early January?

Mr Seymour: At least seven or eight pounds. I was right off my
food; it was a struggle to eat anything.

Dr Johnston: And you said you were very worried that it might be
cancer. Just how worried were you at that point,
between December and early January?

Mr Seymour: I couldn't get it out of my head that it might be cancer.
I couldn't get off to sleep through worrying about it. It
was a struggle to keep on working, because I was
beginning to feel tired, as well as worrying about the
cancer.

Dr Johnston: Just how tired were you?

Mr Seymour: I felt exhausted; it was hard to do things around the house.

It can be seen that the use of clarification ('How worried were you?'; 'How tired were you?') was effective in eliciting the true nature of the patient's experience. Such *clarification* should continue until an exact understanding of the nature, intensity, frequency, and duration of the patient's problems has been obtained.

Responding to cues

Clarification is only possible if the interviewer has been alert to cues given by the patient about possible problem areas or further aspects of these. One difficulty is that patients will often mention several problems at once. There is then a danger that the health professional will selectively attend to a particular cue and ignore the others:

Mr Wallace: How have you been since I saw you last time?

Mrs Taylor: My arm is just as swollen and painful. I find it difficult to comb my hair. I am finding it difficult to cope with my chores, especially as I seem to be increasingly tired. However, my wound seems to be healing up nicely.

Mr Wallace: I am pleased about the wound; but clearly your arm is still giving you trouble. Let me have a look at you.

The cue about Mrs Taylor's feeling increasingly tired is missed, and is not raised again in the consultation. Let us look at what could have happened had Mr Wallace picked up the cue:

Mr Wallace: How have you been since I last saw you?

Mrs Taylor: My arm is still painful and swollen. I have great difficulty doing my hair. I am finding it difficult to cope with my day-to-day chores, particularly as I am getting increasingly tired, although my wound is healing nicely since I had the antibiotics.

Mr Wallace: OK, you have mentioned problems with your arm, but I am pleased to hear your wound is healing nicely. I'll check about your arm in a minute; but you also mentioned feeling tired. Just what's been happening?

Mrs Taylor: It is such an effort to get up and do things. At times I can't be bothered, I feel so miserable.

Mr Wallace: Can you tell me more about this feeling of being miserable?

Mrs Taylor: I burst into tears for no reason. I keep thinking I'm going to die from the cancer. I can't get to sleep for worrying about it.

By ensuring that he paid attention to each of the cues that Mrs Taylor gave, Mr Wallace has elicited the fact that she is developing symptoms of severe depression.

Responding to cues that might suggest psychological problems, particularly cues about emotional distress, is especially important in promoting patient disclosure. It affects disclosure across all domains, including physical, social, psychological, and spiritual issues. Clarifying psychological cues also makes it much more likely that the patient will disclose and express associated feelings.

However alert an interviewer is, it is difficult to keep track of the many cues that the patient may give. It is, therefore, important to note the cues down. Far from inhibiting disclosure, this will indicate to the patient that the key messages are being recorded. The cues can be ticked off notes once they have been properly clarified, and outstanding cues can be checked and dealt with later.

There is often the belief that all cues should be picked up immediately. In fact it is very common to miss certain cues, especially if several are given at the same time. This should not cause concern, since most patients will repeat the cue until it is picked up or until they realize that the health professional is ignoring the message.

Questions with a psychological focus

In addition to open directive questions which focus on patients' perceptions of their diseases and reactions to it, it is important to ask open questions about the impact of the disease on the patient, as was discussed in Chapter 3. Without such an explicit focus patients may withhold important information about the effect of the illness and disease on their lives.

Dr Johnston: What effect has all this had on you in yourself apart from causing you worry?

Mr Seymour: Despite being so tired I managed to stay at work until the operation. My family have been very supportive. However, I have been too tired to pursue my usual hobbies like golf, and I have been unable to do things around the house.

Dr Johnston:	Has it had any effect on your relationships within the family?
Mr Seymour:	No, my wife has been very understanding, and just concerned that there would be treatment to get me better. The two children have been put in the picture and are taking it well. So I have no worries on that score.
Dr Johnston:	You've mentioned being worried and anxious, and say you're feeling more confident now. Has all this led you at any stage to become particularly miserable or depressed?
Mr Seymour:	No, not at all.

Note that in addition to the open questions, Dr Johnston has asked an important question about the patient's mood, since it is common for patients to feel both anxious and depressed in such a predicament, and to develop an anxiety state and/or depressive illness.

In many assessments the story is relatively straightforward. However, the situation can require much more exploration of particular problems and feelings. Here, the difficulty is to know how long to continue exploring one problem before moving on to the next.

Encouraging the expression of emotions

Effective interviewing which includes exploring how patients have reacted to their diagnosis and treatment will lead many patients to disclose that they have been feeling distressed. This emotional distress will be obvious from their tone of voice or from their bursting into tears. It is important to encourage them to express their distress promptly and constructively, providing they are willing to do so.

Dr Paterson:	How did you feel when you heard you had cancer? [open question]
Mrs Taylor:	Terrified.
Dr Paterson:	In what way terrified? [clarification]
Mrs Taylor:	I kept seeing myself in a coffin.
Dr Paterson:	That sounds awful for you. [empathy]
Mrs Taylor:	It was. It was terrible.
Dr Paterson:	I can see you are becoming very distressed. [acknowledgement]
Mrs Taylor:	Yes, it is very upsetting to think about it.
Dr Paterson:	Can you bear to talk about this image of yourself being in a coffin? [negotiation]

Mrs Taylor:	Yes, though I know it will upset me.
Dr Paterson:	Why do you equate having cancer with being in a coffin?
Mrs Taylor:	My mother and elder sister both died from it.
Dr Paterson:	Are there any other reasons why you are so upset when you think of the coffin, other than your knowledge that your mother and elder sister died of it? [exploring reasons]
Mrs Taylor:	I thought I could fight the cancer; but when I read in a magazine that Jill Ireland had died despite her best efforts, it made me feel like giving up. I felt the cancer would just sweep over me.
Dr Paterson:	Any other reasons why you're distressed?
Mrs Taylor:	No.
Dr Paterson:	Just how distressed have you been?
Mrs Taylor:	At times I felt I was at breaking-point. I have not been able to get the images of coffins out of my mind.

By acknowledging Mrs Taylor's distress, being empathic, negotiating, and moving on to explore the component reasons and prompting her to describe these the patient was allowed to express her distress fully, but to move on without getting to a position where she would be hard to rescue. Further aspects of handling distress are discussed in the chapter on handling difficult situations (Chapter 7).

Using silence

There is a skill in using silence, for many distressed individuals find it difficult to articulate their feelings. It is tempting to fill the gap, rather than to give a patient time and space.

Dr Paterson:	Just how distressed have you been?
Mrs Taylor:	[Silence]
Dr Paterson:	For instance, have you cried a lot?

In the above exchange, Dr Paterson filled the silence with his own perceptions, rather than waiting as follows:

Dr Paterson:	Just how distressed have you been?
Mrs Taylor:	[Silence; then] At times I felt at breaking-point.

If silences last too long they carry the risk that patients will become increasingly upset and emotionally disorganized, because they feel overwhelmed by their worries. So, it is crucial to maintain a reasonable momentum.

What Dr Paterson could have done was to acknowledge the silence and its cause.

Mrs Taylor: [Silence]
Dr Paterson: You seem to be finding this quite difficult.
Mrs Taylor: Yes, it is hard to find the words.

Commonly, health professionals respond to distress by reflecting back the last words that the patient has used. This, if continued, can leave the patient feeling 'stranded' and overwhelmed by feelings. Acknowledging the difficulty can help to 'move the patient on' to express their feelings.

Patients do not always admit to being distressed, but the health professional may have a feeling that the patient *is* upset. This feeling should be shared, since it shows a willingness to 'get alongside' the patient in her predicament (*making an educated guess*).

Nurse Menzies: As we talk, I get the feeling you are much more upset than you are letting on.
Mrs Smith: Yes, I suppose I have to admit that it has really shaken me up.
Nurse Menzies: How shaken up have you felt?
Mrs Smith: To be honest, I am terrified; but I don't like to admit it.

Even if the guess is not followed by such elaboration or is repudiated by the patient, it still has a positive effect on disclosure.

Emotional level of the interview
One of the therapeutic functions of an assessment interview is to allow those patients who wish it to have the opportunity to identify and express the feelings associated with their predicament, whether about the diagnosis or about the treatment or other consequences. It is, therefore, important that the interviewer should know how to assess the emotional level of the interview as it proceeds. This can be done by using a four-point scale, in which 0 = there is no hint, mention, or expression of feelings; 1 = merely hints of feelings; 2 = mention, but no expression of feeling; and 3 = mention and expression of feelings. Using the techniques discussed in the chapter on handling distress (Chapter 7), the interviewer is trying to encourage the patient into and out of level 3 in relation to the key problems disclosed (Faulkner 1992).

Handling transitions

In the following interview the patient revealed early on that she found it hard to adapt to the loss of the breast following a mastectomy for breast cancer. She also had severe adverse effects during a course of combination adjuvant chemotherapy, especially sickness. The problem for the interviewer is to know how far to explore each of these issues before moving on to the next topic. The key question the interviewer should ask is 'Have I elicited sufficient information about the nature and extent of the problem and associated feelings to have a reasonable understanding of how it must have been for the patient?' Before exploring a patient's reactions to key treatment events it is important first to *negotiate* whether she is prepared to talk about it. Some patients will find it too painful. To insist on their talking about it then increases their emotional distress, and may hinder their adaptation. However, the majority of patients will feel better for having shared their experiences and expressed their feelings with somebody who appears to understand what it was like. Such understanding can best be demonstrated by the use of *empathic statements*, as shown below.

Sister Morgan: You say your mastectomy really shook you up: can you bear to tell me about that?

Mrs Holroyd: I felt lopsided, repulsive, a freak. I no longer felt a woman, I didn't feel I would ever be attractive to anyone again. I can't even bear to look at myself now. I feel so self-conscious in the company of other people. I feel sure somehow that they can guess that I have lost a breast.

Sister Morgan: So; surgery devastated you then. [empathy]

Mrs Holroyd: Yes, somehow I don't think I will ever feel like a woman again.

Sister Morgan: Has this had any other effects on you apart from those you have just described?

Mrs Holroyd: No, I don't think so.

At this point Sister Morgan feels she has a reasonable grasp of how the mastectomy has affected Mrs Holroyd in respect of her body image; but she wants to check whether it has affected her relationship with her partner. So, she asks an open directive question.

Sister Morgan: How has having had a mastectomy affected your relationship with your partner?

Mrs Holroyd: He has been very loving. He tells me that I am the same woman he married and that my only having one breast doesn't affect him. I find that hard to believe. I can't accept it. I no longer get any enjoyment out of love-making, although I put up with it for his sake.

Sister Morgan then asks a further *screening question* about whether there have been any other problems associated with the mastectomy; but Mrs Holroyd says there have not. She, therefore, feels that it is appropriate to move on, but checks before doing so.

Sister Morgan: So: really your mastectomy has devastated you and had quite a serious effect on how you feel about yourself in relation to your partner. It has made you feel very self-conscious. Do you feel I have got a reasonable grasp of how it has affected you?

Mrs Holroyd: Yes, you have.

Sister Morgan: Is it all right, then, if I move on to ask you about the chemotherapy?

Mrs Holroyd: Yes, that was even worse.

Sister Morgan: So, could you bear to tell me just what happened?

Mrs Holroyd: I was terribly sick after each treatment; I would vomit for two to three days, couldn't eat anything, and became increasingly worried about further treatment.

Sister Morgan then establishes the exact nature of these adverse effects, and then screens for other problems. It becomes clear that the patient has had a bad experience of chemotherapy, and is very reluctant to have more.

Transitions may be initiated by patients when they feel that a sequence is complete. However, patients may introduce important topics *before* the previous topic has been fully explored. In this event, the health professional needs to acknowledge what has been said, and to negotiate the completion of the existing topic.

Sister Morgan: So: chemotherapy was a terrible time for you, then?

Mrs Holroyd: Yes, it was. I got so low I began to feel life wasn't worth living.

Sister Morgan: So you clearly felt very down, then? Can I share a problem with you?

Mrs Holroyd: Yes.

Sister Morgan: You mentioned feeling so low you didn't feel life was worth living. What I would like to do is to continue with your history and then come back to that. Is that all right?

Mrs Holroyd: Yes.

Mrs Holroyd might have insisted that Sister Morgan take a history of what sounds to have been a depressive illness. However, most patients will stay in sequence, providing they know the nurse or other health professional will return to the new topic at some stage during the assessment or on a subsequent occasion.

Summary

In carrying out a basic assessment it is important to promote the use of positive behaviours (open directive questions, eliciting and clarifying psychological and social aspects, summarizing, empathy, and educated guesses), by using relevant skills. It is also important to emphasize the value of negotiation, of helping the patient stay in sequence, and of managing transitions.

It is also important to remember that, unless one is simply seeking facts, closed questions may inhibit disclosure, as may leading questions and inappropriate advice and reassurance.

References

Faulkner, A. (1992). *Effective interaction with patients.* Churchill Livingstone, Edinburgh.

5

Breaking the news to patients

Once a diagnosis of cancer seems possible or certain the doctor or nurse has to determine how much a patient wishes to know about his or her diagnosis, investigation, and treatment. This has to be done in a way that facilitates psychological adaptation and ensures compliance with advice and treatment.

Explaining the diagnosis

It has been found that one of the best predictors of patients' ability to adapt psychologically to the news that they have cancer and require treatment for it is that they should perceive the information they have been given as adequate to their needs (Fallowfield *et al.* 1990). The key task for the health professional, therefore, is to establish a patient's information needs, rather than making assumptions about whether or not she or he is the kind of person who wants the truth or prefers not to know.

How the news about diagnosis is given depends on the patient's awareness of what is likely to be wrong. The level of the patient's awareness should have been established using the methods discussed in Chapters 3 and 4 on initial assessment. The majority of patients with cancer are aware that they could have cancer at the time of investigation. It is then a matter of confirming that their perceptions are correct.

Patients who have no idea that they have cancer pose a particular problem. For it is unclear whether they want to know the whole truth, a partial truth, or nothing. Telling them bluntly that they have cancer carries a high risk that they will deny the news or become overwhelmed with distress. The health professional, therefore, has to have a way of 'testing the waters' to decide how much a patient wishes to know about his or her disease (Maguire and Faulkner 1988).

In this example, enquiry about a patient's perceptions of what is wrong reveals that she has no idea that she has cancer of the ovary.

| Nurse Jones: | You tell me you have had this pain in your tummy for a few weeks. You have lost a lot of weight and you have been feeling very tired. Have you any thoughts as to what it might be? |
| Mrs Avery: | The only thing I can think of is a grumbling appendix. |

The nurse now has to attempt to change the patient's perception of having a grumbling appendix to the reality of having ovarian cancer. She can best do this by giving a clear warning that the condition is serious ('I can understand you think it might be a grumbling appendix, but I'm afraid it looks more serious.').

The nurse should then pause and give the patient time to respond, rather than rushing on and giving the cancer diagnosis. For this would provoke denial or emotional disorganization, because the transition from the perception of being well to that of having a potentially fatal illness would then be too abrupt.

A minority of patients will indicate that they have no wish to acquire any more information, by saying, for example, 'I don't really want to know any more than that. I take it you can do something to treat it?' Their wishes should be respected.

When the patient wishes to know what is meant by 'serious', it is worth taking her a step further and explaining that the investigations showed that it might be 'a kind of tumour'. This use of euphemisms allows the health professional to proceed from giving a warning through a hierarchy of euphemisms until she gets to the point where the patient pulls out or indicates she wishes to hear that it is 'cancerous'. ('What do you mean a kind of tumour?'). Alternatively, the patient may anticipate the disclosure, and say 'So: it is cancer, then?' It is particularly import-ant to avoid forcing information upon those patients who indicate that they do not wish to have detailed information about their disease or prognosis. They will usually still want information about treatment, and will comply with its indications.

When the patient indicates she wants to go through the full truth-telling process, and is given the bad news that she has cancer, it is important that the nurse pauses to give the woman time to assimilate the information and think about its implications. This is hard to do in practice, because health professionals wish to try to soften the bad news by giving the patient some encouraging information. However, if the nurse moves into reassurance and advice mode ('I know it's bad news you have got cancer; but the good news is we can cure it and get you better in no time') the patient will still be assimilating the bad news and worrying about it. Consequently, she will not take in much of the offered advice or reassurance. Indeed, she is likely only to remember any negative phrase used by the nurse (for example, 'There could be some residual cells'), and ignore any positive information. The nurse should first acknowledge and explore the patient's distress.

Acknowledging the distress

It is important that the health professional is not frightened by the distress that inevitably emerges if bad news is given effectively. For it is bound to be upsetting. So the first step is to acknowledge this distress by saying 'I can see the news that I have given you has distressed you greatly. Could you bear to say why?' This explicit invitation to talk about her distress and its underlying reasons legitimizes for the patient the process of doing so.

Dr Peters: I'm sorry to have had to tell you that it's cancer. I can see it has upset you.

Mrs Molloy: I'm devastated.

Dr Peters: Can you bear to tell me about it?

Mrs Molloy: It's the one thing I dreaded. My mother died of cancer, and my daughter is due to get married in a few months' time. It couldn't have come at a worse time.

Dr Peters: I can understand that. Are there any other reasons why you are feeling so distressed?

It then helps if the doctor or nurse summarizes the patient's concerns, checks if there are other concerns, explores these, and discusses with the patient whether she would like information about further investigations and treatment:

Dr Peters: Your main concern seems to be that the cancer has come at a rotten time for you in view of your daughter's getting married. It has reminded you of your mother's death from cancer and made you very fearful about your own future. No wonder you feel so distressed. Are there any other issues that concern you at the moment?

Mrs Molloy: No, only that something can be done to treat it.

Once a list of the patient's concerns provoked by the bad news has been elicited it is important to decide in what order to discuss them with the patient. As time may be short, it is helpful to summarize them and ask the patient to put them in order of priority, unless there is an overriding medical problem. This ensures that the main problems can be dealt with even if there is insufficient time to deal with less important ones:

Nurse Spry: As I understand it your main concern is not so much the cancer, because they are going to be able to remove all of it, but the fact you are going to need a colostomy. You are worried about its leaking and affecting your social life and personal relationships.

Mrs Bond: Yes, that's correct.

Nurse Spry: Do you have any other worries at the moment?

Mrs Bond: Isn't that enough?

Nurse Spry: Well, it's important to check I haven't missed anything before we discuss what we might be able to do.

Mrs Bond: All right.

Nurse Spry: Which of these concerns is bothering you the most?

Mrs Bond: Having to try and cope with the colostomy.

Nurse Spry: So shall we begin, then, by talking about what we might be able to do to try and help you with that?

Mrs Bond: Yes, I would be grateful if you would.

Notice here that the nurse talks about 'trying to help', as opposed to promising that she will be able to help. In this way she has pitched her helpful statement at the right level, so that it will promote hope without leading to false expectations.

Checking understanding

Once information has been given about diagnosis and treatment in a clear way it is important that the health professional checks with the patient that she has understood what has been said. However well the bad news has been broken and the information has been given the patient may not take it all in correctly, so this checking is important.

Another way of giving patients opportunities to reconsider the information given and to check it is to invite them to have a companion present when the bad news is broken, or to take home a tape-recording of the consultation (Hogbin *et al.* 1992).

Questions about prognosis

When bad news is broken it is likely to provoke questions about the eventual prognosis of the cancer. It is best to try to pitch the answer to this at an appropriate level. Thus, when there is a good prospect of cure the doctor might say 'There is every hope we can cure it at this stage.'

However, if the prognosis is less clear it is important to indicate this by saying 'We are reasonably hopeful that we can cure it.' When the outlook looks more bleak appropriate phrases might include 'We should be able to control it' or 'I don't think we are going to be able to cure it, but I do think we can relieve some of those symptoms, particularly the pain you have been suffering.' Such statements about prognosis may provoke further distress and new concerns. So these should then be explored and understood, and appropriate reassurance and advice should be offered.

It is important to try to avoid being pressured by patients or relatives to give precise predictions about how long the patient will live. If you are forced to give an indication it is best to phrase this in terms of months or years, rather than giving an exact date. When patients have important life decisions to make and it is unclear that they are going to respond to treatment it is better to advise them to err on the side of caution, and to make a decision rather than leaving it.

Dr Thomas:	How has the news left you feeling?
Mr McDonald:	Shocked. It couldn't have come at a worse time.
Dr Thomas:	How do you mean?
Mr McDonald:	I am just about to buy a second home. We have planned it for so long.
Dr Thomas:	So this news has been especially disappointing?
Mr McDonald:	Yes: I'm not sure what to do, whether to press ahead or not.
Dr Thomas:	As I explained, your tumour should respond to treatment, but I cannot be sure until we have tried it. So, in these circumstances, perhaps you should postpone your decision until we know how you are responding. Is that possible?
Mr McDonald:	I think others will snap it up if we don't. Yet if anything happens to me, my wife will be left with a big financial burden.
Dr Thomas:	That's a hard decision to make, then?

Once the patient has taken on board the diagnosis and likely outcome in terms of treatment, it is useful to discuss in more detail the possible treatment available.

Treatment choices
There is some evidence (Morris and Royle 1988) that patients who are offered a choice of treatment (when this is technically possible) cope

better than those who are not given any options, providing they are the kind of patients who want to be involved in choice instead of leaving it to the treating clinician. So it is important to check out whether patients have any particular views about the treatment options available, and to follow their wishes whenever possible. Such a policy seems to also affect the partner's psychological adaptation favourably.

In helping patients formulate their choice of treatment it is important to let them carry out a decision analysis. This involves the patients' generating the positive reasons for adopting each treatment and the negative reasons for rejecting it before doing the same for any other alternative treatment. They can then scan the lists of reasons. They can only do this exercise properly if they have had adequate information about the nature and possible adverse effects of the different treatments. It is important to give them honest information, so that they are not falsely reassured that a treatment, such as for example combination chemotherapy, is relatively mild when it might cause major adverse effects, and so lead to the patients' becoming bitter and distrustful.

When patients are parents they may well ask whether they should inform their children.

Facilitating psychological adaptation

Once the patient has assimilated the fact that he has cancer he has to cope with several major psychological hurdles if he is to adapt. These include how to cope with the uncertainty of prognosis; a search for an explanation of why he has developed cancer; whether there is anything he can do to contribute towards his survival; how open to be about his predicament with friends, relatives, and employers; and how to obtain emotional and practical support. There is also an issue about whether knowing he has cancer has caused him to feel stigmatized by it or to worry about the reaction of other people towards him. So it is crucial that the doctor or nurse following up the patient should ask specific questions within a few weeks of the cancer diagnosis being given.

- How do you see your illness working out?
- Have you any theories about why you have got cancer?
- Is there anything you feel you can do to combat your illness and contribute to your survival?
- Have you been able to be open to people close to you about what has happened?
- How much support do you feel you have been getting from close friends and family since your illness was diagnosed?

- Has having had cancer diagnosed affected how you feel about yourself in any way?
- How much support do you feel you have been getting from your doctors and the nurses who are looking after you?

If patients have not dealt with these hurdles they are likely to develop an anxiety state or a depressive illness. So it is important to try and help them overcome them.

Relapse

The time of first relapse can be especially distressing for a cancer patient who had come to believe that he or she was cured or would survive for some years. Here, the same principles about breaking bad news apply. Thus, the patient's own awareness should be checked. The health professional should 'test the waters' in the way described earlier, in order to be able to determine how much information patients know or are ready for.

There is then the challenge of helping them cope with the uncertainty.

Handling uncertainty

Some patients are able to put worry about what will happen to them to the back of their minds. They accept the news that they have a recurrence without becoming unduly upset. However, the majority will be greatly worried that the cancer has recurred, that they may suffer a premature death but face an inevitable uncertainty about how and when this may occur.

It is important to check if the patient is finding this uncertainty hard to manage by asking, 'How do you see things working out?'. It is important to acknowledge that the uncertainty is a real problem. ('You are right. We can't be sure at this stage how things are going to work out. This must be hard for you?'). It is useful to check if patients would like detailed information about the current status of their disease and the subsequent effects of treatment; just wish to be given general information; or prefer not to know.

It also helps to ask those patients who wish to have full information if they would like to know what symptoms might herald a further recurrence once treatment has brought this episode under control. These marker symptoms should be explained and the patient should be advised to get in touch immediately should any such symptoms develop between appointments. Most patients will view the absence of these symptoms as a good sign and cope well.

Most patients welcome regular follow-up but some need more frequent appointments because the reassurance of a check-up wears off after only a few weeks. Hence, it is worth asking patients how they feel about the frequency of follow-ups and whether it is meeting their psychological as well as physical needs.

Terminal care

Inevitably, for some cancer patients there comes a point when active treatment is no longer possible. Again, it is a matter of checking their awareness. If they realize that their cancer cannot be cured it is important to confirm that, and then explore the resultant concerns.

Dr Brown:	You say you have been very tired and having terrible pain in your back. What have you been making of all this?
Mr Vernon:	The treatment is clearly not working any more.
Dr Brown:	I'm afraid you're right, it isn't.
Mr Vernon:	Is there anything else you can do?
Dr Brown:	I'm afraid not. We have reached the end of the line as far as active treatment is concerned. I am sorry to have to tell you that.
Mr Vernon:	I think I had realized that anyway.
Dr Brown:	How does that leave you feeling?
Mr Vernon:	Well, I'm resigned to it in many ways. I have had a good innings and a good life. What I am really concerned about is I don't suffer too much.
Dr Brown:	Why is that?
Mr Vernon:	My father died of lung cancer. He wasted away in front of me, and had terrible pain despite everybody's efforts.
Dr Brown:	Well, that's something we will try and do our best to avoid if we possibly can, by keeping a close eye on you and trying to help you. Any other concerns?
Mr Vernon:	No.

Other patients may indicate a lack of awareness, and wish to deny the gravity of their illness. It is important to respect this unless there are compelling reasons to challenge it.

Some patients oscillate in and out of awareness and denial, and so it is important to check their awareness repeatedly during subsequent consultations so as to avoid making assumptions about how much information they want.

Challenging denial

Sometimes, it is necessary to challenge denial because patients may have some important unfinished business to conduct or because they are refusing a treatment which might alleviate symptoms. It is important to be able to confront denial in a way that maximizes the possibility of breaking it without causing psychological harm.

In the following example, a man with an 'apparent ulcer' had a laparotomy which showed him to have widespread metastatic bowel cancer, with no prospect of a response to active treatment. The surgeon had been unable to remove any of the tumour, and went along a day later to see the patient in a side-room off the ward.

Mr Johns:	How are you feeling today?
Mr Smithers:	Very sore; it hurts when I cough.
Mr Johns:	How are you feeling otherwise?
Mr Smithers:	Fine, absolutely fine. I am confident you have killed it.
Mr Johns:	What makes you think that?
Mr Smithers:	One of the nurses told me I was in and out of theatre in no time. So it must have been a simple job.
Mr Johns:	Has it crossed your mind that there might be any other explanation for why you spent such a short time in theatre?
Mr Smithers:	No; it has got to be good news, hasn't it?

Here the attempt to confront the wishful thinking has not been successful. So the surgeon should challenge this denial, while avoiding disorganizing the patient emotionally. It is possible that there may be a 'window' on denial, in that for at least some time of each waking day the patient has considered that his prospects are not so good. The surgeon can explore this as follows:

Mr Johns:	So you were pleased when you heard that you were in and out of theatre in a short time, and you haven't considered any other reason for that except that things went very well?
Mr Smithers:	No.
Mr Johns:	Are you sure? Has there been any time since the operation when you have considered that things might not have been so straightforward, even for a few seconds?
Mr Smithers:	Well, yes.
Mr Johns:	Could you bear to tell me about that?
Mr Smithers:	Well, late last night I woke up and I suddenly had this panic.

Mr Johns:	Panic?
Mr Smithers:	I suddenly thought was it because there was nothing you could do that I was in and out so quickly, and then I dismissed that. I thought I was just being stupid.
Mr Johns:	What if it were that we got you in and out of theatre so quickly because we couldn't do anything about your illness.
Mr Smithers:	That would be very hard to bear.
Mr Johns:	Can you bear to think about it for a moment?
Mr Smithers:	[Becoming upset] I guess I have been kidding myself. It has to be serious, hasn't it?
Mr Johns:	I'm afraid so.

Here, checking for a window on denial has been successful. However, when this confirms that the patient is in total denial it is best to leave the patient in that defence mode, and wait for a further opportunity as the illness progresses. For many patients are unable to maintain denial once their disease progresses beyond a certain point. This may even be within a day or so of death. It is important to be vigilant for the opportunity, because this allows the health professional to check out with the patient whether there are important areas of unfinished business, both practically and emotionally, that they have yet to deal with. Doing this should prevent some of the major problems associated with unresolved grief (Chapter 11).

It is important to avoid confronting denial aggressively. For denial is a necessary defence when the patient finds it intolerable to consider the reality. Stripping away denial aggressively may intensify denial or cause overwhelming distress, which can lead to an anxiety state or depressive illness.

A woman with two children who was married to an effective and supportive partner was dying of a brain tumour. She kept insisting that it was benign and that she would recover. This frustrated both her husband and the health professionals involved in her care. Consequently, a social worker was summoned and asked to challenge her denial. She did repeatedly confront the patient by saying 'You have to face the fact you have cancer. Your husband and family need to be able to talk to you about important things. As long as you continue to deny things this makes it very difficult for them.'

This patient responded by getting very angry and throwing a plant pot at the social worker, which hit her in the face.

A few days later, when she realized her disease was progressing, she was able to accept the reality of her disease. She was able to have important discussions with her husband and children which relieved a lot of the unfinished business and associated distress.

Some patients are left with falsely optimistic views of their illness because they have been misled deliberately. Here the difficulty lies in deciding how to deal with this misinformation.

The misinformed patient

When questions are asked about the patient's awareness it becomes apparent that their level of awareness is linked to their having been given falsely optimistic information about the extent of their disease and its likely prognosis. The task for the health professional is to try to help them adopt a more appropriate perception without disorganizing them emotionally.

The same principles which were advocated for breaking bad news should be followed:

Sister Edwards: How do you see things working out?

Mr Owen: Very well. They assured me that they had got rid of the lung tumour first time around. They told me that I should live out a reasonable life-span.

Sister Edwards: But you are back in here with this bad dry cough of yours, and you have been losing weight: is that right?

Mr Owen: Yes, but I am still confident that everything is sorted.

Sister Edwards: I am afraid things look more serious than that.

Mr Owen: What on earth do you mean?

Sister Edwards: I'm afraid I don't think your illness has responded as well as they said.

Mr Owen: What exactly do you mean? [indicating a wish to hear the information]

Sister Edwards: It looks like it's returned.

Mr Owen: Why on earth couldn't they tell me the truth? They have really let me down in a big way.

Sister Edwards: I really don't know. They may have had good reasons for protecting you from what was happened; but the fact we have to face now is what is actually happening.

Mr Owen: I suppose in some way I should be grateful to you for that; but I feel so angry that they didn't put me in the picture in the first place.

It is hard to impart an accurate prognosis to a patient, because the course of the disease can be so unpredictable, particularly when the disease has recurred. This can result in some patients living on 'borrowed time'.

Living on borrowed time

Here the health professional is likely to be encountered by a patient who is angry that he or she is dying much sooner than was predicted, or living longer. It is important to acknowledge his or her feelings, explore the reasons for them, and establish a constructive relationship.

Dr Forbes: You seem very angry?

Mr Booth: I'm furious.

Dr Forbes: Why?

Mr Booth: I feel very angry about what the doctors said to me.

Dr Forbes: How do you mean?

Mr Booth: They said I would live at least two years, and now it's less than six months, and I know I am going downhill.

Dr Forbes: Yes, I'm afraid it looks like it.

Mr Booth: Well, thinking I had at least two years I made lots of plans, and I postponed other decisions that I ought to have taken about disposing of my business assets.

Dr Forbes: What makes you so angry?

Mr Booth: They were so confident that I would be well and live a reasonable length of time. If they had admitted they were uncertain I could have reacted very differently.

Dr Forbes: I can understand your feeling angry about that. But it can be very difficult to predict how people will respond to treatment with this kind of illness.

Mr Booth: Yes, I accept that; but it doesn't alter the fact that I have wasted a lot of time when I could have been getting on with things. Now I am beginning to feel too weak and tired to do all the things I wanted.

Dr Forbes: Would it be worth our sitting down and just discussing what they might be in the hope we might be able to help you do at least some of them.

Mr Booth: I suppose so.

Summary

Matching the information given about a patient's illness and treatment to what the patients wish to know and are ready to know can help in a major way to facilitate their adaptation to their predicaments, regardless of the stage of disease. The key is to be flexible and responsive to the individual patient's needs, and to avoid situations where the patient is deliberately misinformed and given either too severe or too optimistic a prognosis.

References

Fallowfield, L. J., Hall, A., Maguire, G. P., and Baum, M. (1990). Psychological outcomes of different treatment policies in women with early breast cancer outside a clinical trial. *British Medical Journal*, **301**, 575–80.

Hogbin, B., Jenkins, V. A., and Parkin, A. J. (1992). Remembering "bad news" consultations. *Psycho-oncology*, **1**, 147–54.

Maguire, P. and Faulkner, A. (1988). How to do it: communicate with cancer patients: 1. Handling bad news and difficult questions. *British Medical Journal*, **297**, 907–9.

Morris, J. and Royle, G. T. (1988). Offering patients a choice of surgery for early breast cancer: a reduction in anxiety and depression in patients and their husbands. *Social Science and Medicine*, **26**, 583–5.

6

Monitoring progress

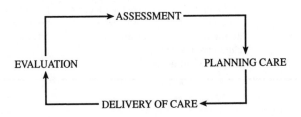

Fig. 6.1 Assessment as part of a dynamic process.

Assessment is not a 'one-off' activity carried out only when the patient is first seen, but is a dynamic ongoing activity, which allows progress to be monitored.

Soon after admission, the patient's problems should have been identified, and their care planned in the light of the presenting problems, whether these are physical, social, or psychological. The patient will still be attempting to come to terms with the illness and its sequelae and treatment, which can be frightening and unpleasant. Fears and worries do not disappear overnight, and nursing and medical staff will need to review both social and psychological problems.

Mary Jackson, for example found a lump in her breast while on holiday. She subsequently had a biopsy followed by a mastectomy. Table 6.1 shows the problems identified a few days after the operation for mastectomy.

The care planned for Mary Jackson dealt with the physical problems of pain and swelling in the left arm, and the social problems, which were possibly more a concern than a reality; and a dialogue was started that allowed Mary to talk through her psychological concerns and to generate some ideas as to how she might deal with them, for example:

Mary:	Will I ever feel the same?
Nurse:	The same?
Mary:	Well, look at me—a lopsided freak. [starts crying]
Nurse:	Can you bear to tell me how you are feeling about that?

Table 6.1 Problems identified following left-side mastectomy on Mary Jackson

Physical	Social	Psychological	Spiritual
Pain at site of scar Swelling in arm (L)	Worried about teenage son (rather wild); husband 'workaholic', seems to resent giving time to child care and hospital visiting.	Worried that husband will no longer love her without breast. Fears her cancer hasn't been eradicated.	Feels loss of control over life events. Sees cancer as a punishment (did not reveal 'crime').

In the ensuing exchange, it was obvious that Mary was at risk of quite severe body-image problems, and also having difficulties in maintaining her beliefs about herself as a 'good' person, and had started worrying that she was being punished (with cancer) for an incident in her adolescence of which she was ashamed.

By the time Mary went home her pain was under control, the swelling in her arm was reducing, and relative harmony was restored in the family. Once Mary and her husband had been able to talk through the worries of her illness intruding on his very busy workload, Jack had been able to reassure Mary. His seeming resentfulness was not that he had to give time to his teenage son, whom he was getting to know rather better than before, but was due to acute worry on his part because his own mother had died of cancer. He had a certain amount of guilt, believing that the people he loved would all get cancer, and that there was a grave risk that he would lose Mary.

What were not resolved on Mary's discharge were her psychological problems. Her husband was being extremely loving, but Mary hadn't shown him her wound, and was still very shy about her operation. She also was feeling under her arms, quite constantly wondering if cancer had spread from the breast to other places. Although there was no talk about it she also appeared to continue to feel some sense of responsibility for her present situation. For these reasons, Mary was asked to agree to see a psychiatrist, as nursing staff felt that more expert help was required.

The ideal in terms of monitoring Mary's progress, or indeed the progress of any patient, would be that the person who did the first assessment would then follow on and be able to check progress on decisions that had been made in negotiation with Mary against the outcomes that had been predicted. In fact this is rarely possible, but what *is* possible is that the first assessor, usually a hospital nurse or doctor, can pass on the relevant information to someone in the community, either the general practitioner or one of the community nurses. Faulkner (1984) found that although a discharge letter is sent to the general practitioner there is little referral of cancer patients into the community nursing service. This makes monitoring a patient difficult, and sometimes impossible, if the district nurses and health visitors are not aware of someone on their patch who has been dis-charged after treatment for cancer.

In Mary Jackson's case she was referred to the district nurse for physical care and monitoring of the swelling in her arm, but the hospital staff had also alerted the district nurse to psychological concerns, the fact that Mary might not have as much support from her husband as she might feel that she needed, and that she was waiting for an appointment with a psychiatrist. In monitoring Mary's progress the district nurse checked out her physical condition, and then had a dialogue about other concerns. She did not assume that Mary's problems were static, but asked her to talk about her problems in adjusting to her current situation. This approach can bring out a new raft of problems, quite different from the ones that arose in hospital, as can be seen below:

District Nurse: Well, Mary, I am pleased to see that your arm is better and that the exercises aren't too painful; it's good that you are doing them so regularly.

Mary: Well, I have got plenty of time: I am not back to work yet.

District Nurse: Are you worried about that?

Mary: Well, it's not that I am worried about it, I know my job's open for me; but I am so bored. I am just not used to being at home all day, and, you know, the exercises—at least it's something to do.

District Nurse: Can you tell me something more about this boredom?

Mary: Well, I suppose I mean lonely. Jack is out of the house soon after seven o'clock, and he often isn't in 'till nine o'clock at night. When I was working it didn't matter. It mattered in hospital, 'cos I thought he wouldn't have time to look after Sam; and it really matters now,

Table 6.2 Problems identified on the monitoring visit: Mary Jackson

Physical	Social	Psychological	Spiritual
Tired. Some pain but better. Can do exercises. Some swelling. Wound well healed.	Husband works 7 a.m.–9 p.m. Son OK. Mary lonely. Friends have not visited.	Sleeping in separate room. Worried about recurrence.	Questioning values. Feels out of control.

because, you know, I have no one. I just long for my friends at work; and at the hospital they said I should see a psychiatrist—and I'm a bit tense waiting for that.

Table 6.2 shows the problems identified by the District Nurse on a visit to monitor Mary's progress. Physical problems were seen to be improving, but there were new problems in both the social and psychological domain. Following assessment, the nurse had to negotiate with Mary to look for solutions to those problems, and to agree a way forward.

Mary agreed to talk to her husband to tell him how much she wanted him to come home a little bit early occasionally to be with her. She also agreed, and it was her suggestion, that she should invite some of her workmates to come and see her. This solution brought up another problem, in that she felt that her workmates might be a little frightened because they knew that she had cancer.

In the psychological domain, there was a sexual problem arising, in that Mary was now sleeping in a separate room from Jack, by her own choice. She had not discussed this with him, and on further questioning admitted that she wasn't quite sure about resuming their sexual life. She was still worried about a recurrence, and, although she no longer talked about cancer as a 'punishment' to the district nurse, she still gave 'vibes' that she was feeling that somehow she was responsible for her own cancer. The nurse, feeling that Mary still had quite a lot of adjusting to do, arranged to check on her appointment with the psychiatrist and to see her in a further two weeks. Between them they set goals for dealing with some of the psychological problems.

Monitoring, then, is necessary at physical, social, and psychological, levels.

Physical adjustment

In monitoring physical adjustment it is important to check out the symptoms prevailing at the time of assessment, and whether they have changed over time, as a result of treatment. Mary Jackson, for example, found that she was very tired when she came home; and this was in contrast to how she felt at the time she found the lump, and had no other very obvious symptoms. If a patient is still under treatment it is necessary to check for side-effects of that treatment. For example, the nausea and vomiting associated with chemotherapy can be modified with suitable treatment; but it is important to have a clear view of exactly how debilitating those side-effects are, and the effect they may be having on physical well-being. Similarly, if the patient has had mutilating surgery, such as a mastectomy or a stoma, then it is necessary to monitor physical adjustment to the surgery. Mary Jackson, for example, could not bear to look at her wound, and was sleeping in a separate room to make sure that her husband didn't see it either.

By monitoring physical adjustment to cancer and its treatment, plans can be made to help further in areas of concern. For example, Mary Jackson was thought to need considerable help to learn to look at her wound and to accept her new body image, so an appointment was made with a psychiatrist. Similarly, a patient with side-effects from chemotherapy may need some treatment to make the regime more acceptable and less invasive of the patient's normal lifestyle. If physical adjustment does not occur then problems can rebound into both social and psychological adjustment. For the nurse or doctor in cancer care it is vital to distinguish between the patient who can be helped by the staff available, and those who need more expert help.

Social adjustment

Social adjustment can be affected by both physical and psychological problems. For example, if patients cannot themselves adjust to the notion of having cancer and the resultant treatment, then it is very likely that their families and friends may also have difficulties. Indeed, in monitoring social adjustment it is quite important to find out how the family has accepted the patient's illness and treatment, and also what effect, if any, this has had on friends.

Mary Jackson was considerably worried about her husband when she was in hospital, in case he did not care adequately for their teenage son. What she had not realized was that her husband was himself very worried about her cancer. When this type of situation occurs, collusion may arise, because the partners themselves can feel so threatened by a diagnosis of cancer that they don't wish to discuss it with their loved ones. This appears to be a protective mechanism motiv-ated by love, and will be considered in Chapter 7.

If the family are not open with each other, then social adjustment is unlikely to take place, since everyone is putting up a wall or barrier of secrecy. In monitoring social adjustment the health professional very often has to deal with worries and concerns of both the patient and family members. This will require negotiation to gain access to people who are concerned but do not necessarily wish to talk about their loved one's cancer.

Similarly with friends, the word 'cancer' is frightening for many people, for many still associate cancer with death. As a result they don't know what to say to a friend diagnosed as having cancer (Buckman 1988), and stalemate can be reached if patients feel that family and friends should be making greater efforts for them.

Effort may be needed from all family members; but patients may not see this if they have not adjusted to their disease and treatment. With Mary Jackson, both her self-image (through her concern that she caused her own cancer) and her body image (in that she feels mutilated) are affected. Until these issues have been dealt with Mary is unlikely to adjust socially to the situation that she had before her illness.

The health professional can identify problems; but the adjustments have to be made by the patients themselves, perhaps with the help of family and friends. This requires, as was seen with Mary Jackson, that the health professional should negotiate with the patient on what action can be taken to deal with current problems. Mary, it will be remembered, was sleeping in a separate room from her husband for psychological reasons; but that in itself could have had some influence on Jack's continuing to work for very long hours, and as a result seeing very little of his wife. This action can be seen as saving him from facing the fact that he has a wife who is now mutilated, and is obviously rejecting him sexually.

It can be seen that social adjustment may take some time, while the patient and her loved ones adjust to changes in many directions. Often patients who enjoyed going out dancing, for meals, and for other social events may well stay in the house much more than before, simply because they no longer feel self-confident enough to meet the rest of the world. Because family members are also very concerned they are not always as helpful as one might hope, and may themselves require help from a health professional to come to terms with the changes in their loved one.

Psychological adjustment

It will have been seen in Chapter 1 that psychological and spiritual concerns are less likely to be disclosed than physical or social concerns. This is equally true when monitoring progress, as on the first assessment. Comparing Table 6.1 with Table 6.2 it can be seen that Mary Jackson's psychological problems remained reasonably constant, even though they were identified.

Mary has dealt with the worry that Jack would no longer love her by simply not being available to her husband. She therefore avoids the issue of whether he loves her or not. Her fear that the cancer will recur has persisted, as has the suggestion that she may be feeling that her cancer is a punishment. If some action is not taken to address these concerns then the patient is very likely to become anxious and perhaps depressed. In monitoring progress it is important to screen for both these reactions to cancer and its treatment, and to refer if more expert help is seen to be required.

The fact of having cancer at all can be a bar to psychological adjustment. Much of Mary Jackson's concerns centred around the diagnosis of cancer and the fear, which appears to be quite common, that having an operation—even a quite traumatic one—does not guarantee that the cancer has gone away. This is a difficult area, since the doctors are not able to assure her that it has. What can be said is that she will be monitored very carefully over the next few years, and that any recurrence will be dealt with immediately; but this is small comfort to many patients who are suffering from cancer.

Similarly with Mary's feelings of guilt. Cancer is often very difficult to explain or understand. Although some cancers are clearly related to lifestyle (witness the link between lung cancer and smoking), many others do not seem to have any such linkage that the average individual can understand. This brings people's beliefs and values about themselves into sharp relief. The senselessness of the situation gives many patients the notion that life events are totally outside their control, and one way for them to make sense of what is happening is to take the 'blame' upon themselves.

The health professional needs to give patients time and space to talk through these concerns, and to negotiate ways in which patients may be enabled to move their thinking forward to a point at which they can rid themselves of guilt.

Similarly with sexual problems, which are not uncommon in cancer patients. Mary Jackson felt that she was no longer attractive to her husband, so when she came home she slept in a separate room, and was quite distant with Jack. He responded by working even longer hours than usual; and so a situation arose where they were living in the same house, but not really meeting as partners.

Many health professionals would argue that this is private and personal between the patient and her husband, and that they have no right to pry. In fact, sexual problems can hamper psychological adjustments to such an extent that if the patient is willing to disclose the problem and consider ways of dealing with it the whole picture can change radically for both partners. This process starts with the professional giving encouragement for the patient to disclose. Mary had to come to grips with her own body image before she could deal with the problem of exposing her extreme vulnerability to her husband.

In monitoring adjustment to cancer and its treatment, a very important question is to ask patients how they view the current situation. This may happen as follows:

District Nurse: Mary, you have obviously got quite a few problems, and we'll talk in a minute about what we might do about those; but what's your overall view of the current situation?

Mary: It all looks a bit black, really: I don't know how Jack and I are ever going to start talking again. I know a lot of it's my fault; but things look pretty grim.

District Nurse: That sounds fairly strong.

Mary: Well, you know, I can't see me ever being back to what I was—and I was so lively. Jack was so proud of me; but he hasn't asked me out since I came home. No dinner, he hasn't brought me flowers, it's as if I don't exist for him any more. Is this psychiatrist going to help?

In the above exchange, even though the nurse had monitored progress and picked up the current problems, she gained more depth of knowledge of Mary's deep anxiety. She is also faced with the patient's concerns about psychiatric intervention.

The important point in reassessment is to look for normal versus abnormal reactions to the current situation. It could be argued, for example, that Mary was not unusual in seeing life in deep and dark terms following mutilating surgery and its aftermath. She may indeed be the sort of person who reacts to most traumas by looking on the absolutely blackest side. This points up a very important issue about both assessment and monitoring. For, if a decision is to be made as to whether a patient is coping or not, then current reactions have to be measured against how that individual normally copes with life crises. What the health professional is looking for is a change from how that patient was before the illness. A useful question is, 'How different are things now from what they were before you knew you were ill?' This gives patients a chance to describe the way they were before and any subsequent changes, for example:

Mary: I suppose I have always been a bit of a Jonah; Jack says that I'd find trouble in any situation.
District Nurse: And is your current reaction along similar lines?
Mary: No, the way I am looking at things at the moment is dark, even for me.

In the above exchange it can be seen that Mary is well aware that she is much more anxious and concerned than she has been in previous difficult situations.

Change can, however, happen in a positive direction. In a study carried out by Maguire and Faulkner (Faulkner 1984) one patient reported that since she had come home from her hospitalization her husband had behaved quite differently from before. She had felt that he took her very much for granted before her cancer, but afterwards he came home with flowers, chocolates, and tickets for a weekend in Paris. Unfortunately these positive changes are less usual than the negative ones.

Looking for change may bring up more problems, particularly that of resentment. Going back to Mary Jackson, she felt that her loneliness was in part due to the fact that friends from work hadn't visited, and a great deal of resentment came out about this. Only by assessment and negotiation did Mary come round to the notion that of course she herself could have invited those friends to visit. The fact was not that they did not care for Mary so much as that they were nervous about what they would say when they saw her (Buckman 1988). This type of dialogue, where patients can suddenly see a way forward, and their own part in current situations, can have a therapeutic effect, even though the objective is to reassess and monitor progress.

Decision-making

In monitoring progress the health professional has to make a decision to assign patients to one of three categories:

1. Is the patient coping, to such an extent that he or she can be left with a telephone number and the responsibility to 'phone if further problems arise?

2. Is the patient likely to cope with some help from the health professional, which requires contracting to make further visits over a period of time and then review?

3. Are patients so disorganized by their disease and its treatment that they need referring for more specialist help?

1. *Coping*

A knowledge of the many and varied problems that patients with cancer may have can lead to the belief that all patients have problems. In fact, many patients cope very well with their disease and its treatment, with the help of a tight and loving social circle. They appear to adapt well to the change in their situation, and over a period of time will report that yes, they are doing things that they were doing before, and may say 'I am not going to let something like cancer ruin my life.' These patients may be left with a telephone number and perhaps (to take a 'belt and braces' approach) with the occasional phone call to see that they are all right.

2. *Some help required*

Many patients find it difficult to deal with their cancer and its treatment, and may not have the support that is so necessary in order for them to talk through problems and look for solutions. Such patients may respond well to a number of visits from a health professional who can monitor their progress and help them to adjust to their new situation. This has to be negotiated with the patient, in order to set times and spaces that are acceptable to both the patient and the health professional, but also, importantly, to lower the risk of the patient becoming dependent on the health professional.

Mary Jackson was at first seen to fall into this second category, because, although she had problems, she was prepared to look at those problems, work on solutions, and move forward. In screening she was not found to be either clinically anxious or depressed. However, she did need a number of visits, and at one point asked that her husband should also be interviewed. This was to help her re-establish the relationship that they had had prior to her illness. In continuing to monitor a patient with problems the decision whether they need referring on can be made at any time. There is a risk, for example, that Mary's black view of the world will become even blacker; and that, together with her body-image problems, was seen as a reason to refer her for more specialist help.

Only by continuing monitoring will the correctness or incorrectness of that decision be made clear.

3. Needs referral

If a patient is found to be clinically anxious or depressed or behaving in such a way as to be in danger, then the health professional needs to refer that patient on to more specialist help. Nurses sometimes have difficulty with this idea, since many have been trained to believe that they have to solve all their patients' problems. What is required from all health professionals is a knowledge of their own limitations in terms of the help that they can give to their patients. If, for example, a patient is clinically depressed, then that patient needs to be assessed by an expert, and his or her depression needs to be treated sooner rather than later. The health professional who ignores this and hopes that 'counselling' will work may run the risk of patients' depressions spiralling downwards, so that they become a danger to themselves in terms of becoming suicidal.

If a patient needs referral then this is normally done through the General Practitioner, and may require some advocacy on the part of the health professional if the general practitioner is unaware of the true nature of the problem. It is not uncommon, for example, for a general practitioner to believe that it is normal to be depressed after mutilating surgery.

This need to convince others of patients' problems is undershored by separating normal levels of anxiety and depression that patients can cope with from abnormal reactions in which patients are totally disorganized by their disease and its treatment. The latter situation then has to be put to a general practitioner in such a way that he or she cannot ignore it, for example by supplying a list of the signs and symptoms that have caused the nurses concern.

Summary

In this chapter the need for monitoring progress and for reassessment has been considered as an ongoing activity for patients with cancer. The need to reassess physical, social, and psychological adjustment after the first assessment has been considered, showing that problems may go away or may change, or new problems may arise. It has been seen that in order to distinguish normal from abnormal reactions there is an obligation to look at problems in terms of change from the patient's normal reactions to trauma. And finally it has been seen that in any monitoring programme the health professional has to make a decision as to whether patients are coping, and need no further help; whether they will cope with the aid of a contract to provide help over a period of time, coupled with reassessment; or whether they will need referring on to more specialized help.

References

Faulkner, A. (1984). Teaching non-specialist nurses assessment skills in the after care of mastectomy patients. Ph.D. thesis, Steinberg collection, RCN, London.

Buckman, R. (1988). *I don't know what to say*. Macmillan, London.

7

Recognizing and handling difficult situations

Many cancer patients have concerns which may pose problems for health professionals, especially when the cause of the concern is not made clear. If difficult situations arise as a result of the patient's, or relatives', fears and worries, it can leave health professionals with the feeling that they are somehow responsible for the patient's emotional state. In this chapter, some difficult situations which commonly occur will be described, and useful strategies for coping with them will be contrasted with less effective, but more common techniques.

All difficult situations are not necessarily engendered by the patient, but a person may give strong cues, which, if recognized, can be used to defuse an otherwise potentially explosive situation. There is a skill in interpreting such cues, both verbal and non-verbal, and in making the ultimate decision as to whether the problem is the patient's or the professional's, in terms of whether any action should be taken. There is also a skill in making a decision on whether to deal with a difficult situation immediately rather than to negotiate for time or referral.

The withdrawn patient
A patient may appear to be withdrawn, in that he does not interact much with other patients or staff. He may spend his time lying in bed looking at the wall, or may retire behind a newspaper or book, showing little interest in what is going on around him. He may prefer to have his meals alone rather than at the communal table. Such a patient may well be a naturally reserved person, who simply does not want to become 'one of the crowd' on the ward, or too friendly with the staff. He may regard eating as social only when he can choose his companions and his environment. If he is coping well with his disease and its treatment, his behaviour is a problem to the staff, because he does not conform to the expectations of a 'good' patient and does not comply with the socialization process encouraged by nurses. Moreover, carrying a tray of

food to his bed may be seen as a chore when other patients eat together at table.

Careful assessment of the patient (Chapters 3 and 4), and of his inter- actions with family and friends, will show if his behaviour is the result of problems which he has difficulty in verbalizing, or is in fact normal for him (Maguire *et al.* 1993*a*). If the behaviour is not within normal limits, it may have an organic cause, or may be due to psychological factors, or to spiritual issues, or to psychiatric morbidity. Screening of anyone who seems to be unhappy (or worse), to the extent that he or she is withdrawing, is mandatory, yet often forgotten as nurses and doctors seek to find solutions to the patient's apparent discomfort. Consider the following exchange:

Nurse: [brightly] Come on, Jack—it may never happen!
Jack: Hmm.
Nurse: There is no need to be so gloomy—we are doing all
             we can. If you would just co-operate—mix a bit—eat
             with the others—you'd find you felt a lot better. It
             isn't all up to us, you know. Now, how about that
             bath?
Jack: [obviously discomfited] All right, Nurse.
Nurse: There, that's better. Doesn't do to dwell on things.

In fact, the above exchange achieves little except that Jack has a bath. The nurse may feel that she has made an effort to get the patient thinking positively, and may feel very frustrated when he subsequently seems even more withdrawn. If she had attempted to assess the situation from Jack's point of view the outcome might have been very different, as the following exchange shows:

Nurse: [gently] You seem very quiet these days, Jack. Do
             you want to talk about it?
Jack: [gruffly] It wouldn't help.
Nurse: Are you sure?
Jack: I'm all right. [pause] Oh, I wish ...
Nurse: What do you wish?
Jack: I wish I'd thought more in the past.
Nurse: Sounds as if you've been doing some serious thinking.
Jack: I have. [long pause then] ... You see, Nurse, I've
             always lived very much from day to day. I've had a
             good job. I didn't have to worry ...
Nurse: And now ...?

Jack: Well, I'm not daft. It's unlikely I'll work again. And I don't know how to tell Judy. She won't manage on her own ...

As the interaction continued, Jack disclosed that he was anxious about his wife's future both financially and emotionally, and blamed himself for not having taken out insurance or encouraged his wife to have more friends, and for not having agreed to the child she so badly wanted to conceive. The nurse could not solve these problems; but by listening in a non-judgemental way she could establish the number, extent, and priority of those problems, and consider intervention alternatives (Chapters 3 and 4). Jack was not naturally withdrawn, and had responded well to the nurse's interest in him.

It may not always be so easy, and considerable patience may be required before the patient's responses become more than monosyllabic; but most people *do* respond to someone who is interested in them and their concerns, especially when there is no attempt to censure the withdrawn behaviour. An open, focused question, asked in a concerned manner, will establish if there is a problem, as with Jack, or if there is not, as in the following:

Nurse: You seem very quiet these days, Jack. Do you want to talk about it?

Jack: To tell you the truth, Nurse, I've always been a bit of a loner. When I first came in there were a lot of things I needed to know, but now ... well, I'm happy with my crosswords.

Nurse: Are you sure? I noticed you even had your lunch on a tray.

Jack: Yes ... well, I've got this problem with my bottom plate. If I eat alone I can take it slowly; and anyway, I'm happy on my own. It's good of you to worry, though.

Such an exchange establishes that Jack is behaving normally without incurring the risk that he will feel criticized. In fact, the reverse is true, since he acknowledges the nurse's concern for him. This is very different from the 'Come on, cheer up' routine, which could anger any patient, whether or not he or she were grappling with seemingly insoluble problems.

The hopeless patient

Often a patient who appears withdrawn may be suffering from feelings of hopelessness and helplessness (Maguire *et al.* 1993*b*). It may be that the diagnosis is known, and the future looks so black that there seems little point in making any effort for a limited future. Appropriate intervention may change a patient's perspective; but the situation is difficult for everyone who is involved with the patient, including relatives and friends, and can be very miserable for the patient, who could become depressed and suicidal.

Again, the most useful first strategy is to acknowledge the patient's apparent misery, and assess the nature and extent of the feelings and their cause. What is *not* useful, but is a common strategy, is to give false hope in an attempt to cheer the patient up or to chide the patient for lack of faith or trust. Jane Mottram felt that she had recovered well from her mastectomy, and so was upset when she received a card to go to hospital for a further course of treatment she had not expected. When, a year later, she had further problems, and was faced with another course of treatment, she suddenly saw the future cut off amid repeated courses of medication that did not work and that made her feel more ill and miserable than her disease. She appeared apathetic, and started talking about the hopelessness of the situation.

Consider the following three approaches to Jane's distress:

A.

Jane: I'm not sure about more treatment—the whole thing is so hopeless I might as well give up now.

Doctor: Come now, Mrs Mottram, how can you think I'd offer you treatment if I didn't believe it would work?

Jane: But the other treatment didn't work.

Doctor: That's pessimistic ... and the new treatment is very good. You'll see—put you right in no time, I'm sure.

B.

Jane: I'm not sure about more treatment—the whole thing is so hopeless I might as well give up now.

Doctor: Look, you can trust me. Don't worry your head about it. Surely you know I'm here to help you.

Jane: But I know I'm getting worse.

Doctor: Now, now! Your job is to have faith in us. It's hard for me if I feel you do not trust me. You have to believe that you are getting better. That is very important to me... to the whole team. You are a special patient, you know. So no more talk of not getting better!

C.

Jane: I'm not sure about more treatment—the whole thing is so hopeless I might as well give up now.

Doctor: What makes you say that?
Jane: Well, it's spreading, isn't it? And it seems so unfair. I
             had my breast off and they said it was all away, and
             then I had that awful treatment. They said it was for
             safety, yet here I am a year later and it's all started up
             again.
Doctor: So you wonder if it's worth it?
Jane: Yes. How can I believe it will be different this time?

In the first two approaches, the reasons for the patient's hopelessness
were not explored; rather she was made to feel guilty for having doubts
and then given false reassurance in A, while in B she was expected to
trust the doctor and to be concerned about the effect on his feelings
when she expressed anxiety. In C, where the patient's feelings were
explored, it was obvious that she was pessimistic because of being
misled in the past about options and outcomes, and had not been
informed or involved in decisions about her care. This information
allowed the doctor to level with her and give realistic markers for the
future both with, and without, treatment. The patient chose the treatment
option, and became more optimistic (though very guardedly), but
without any misconceptions about 'miracle cures'.

Sometimes hopeless patients have no future, and it can be very
difficult to help them find any positive aspects of life to look forward to.
What is often an aim for those who care is that patients reach their
maximum potential within the constraints of their circumstances. However, this may not be realistic for them. The maxim that every cloud has
a silver lining is of little help in a thunderstorm. In such cases, after
careful assessment, it may be necessary to refer the patient to a skilled
counsellor or psychiatrist.

Some patients *may* commit suicide as the only logical step, both to
escape the current situation and to save them from being a burden on
their families. Altruism in this sense is rare. There is then the potential
for a terrible sense of failure for those who have monitored the patient.
If a detailed assessment has been completed, and the patient (as part of
his or her plan) has not disclosed his or her intent, then it should be
possible to accept that in rare cases a patient has made an informed
choice to commit suicide for cogent reasons, even if it does not fit in
with general beliefs on what patient care is all about.

The withdrawn and/or hopeless patient both present potentially difficult situations because they leave us feeling that somehow we should
be restoring them to the role of a 'normal' patient. Hence the efforts to
'cheer them up', which have so little effect. Making assumptions about

what is worrying the patient can also be dangerous, since it leads to solutions being offered which may be totally inappropriate.

In summary, when a patient seems withdrawn, a sensitive assessment has to be made, to establish the cause, before any intervention is attempted. The most usual causes for withdrawal are confusional state, distrust, fear, suppressed anger, feelings of guilt and/or isolation, and psychiatric morbidity, which needs to be referred on.

Other difficult situations may be more explicit. These include overt distress, anger, difficult questions, and patients who want to opt out of treatment or try alternative therapies.

Overt distress

Overt distress seldom occurs in isolation—more usually it is the result of a trigger, and as such can happen at any time. It may, for example, start during assessment, when the patient discusses the feelings surrounding diseases and treatment, and its effect on normal functioning. It may also happen in the ward at visiting time or with other patients; and occasionally distress can be triggered for more obscure reasons, such as when Sister takes the post around and someone who needed a card or a letter as reassurance from a loved one is left out. In such situations the response is emotional, and logic has little place.

No matter when overt distress is encountered, the strategies for handling it are similar. Many professionals find tears difficult to handle because in normal society such raw emotion is either discouraged, or seen as a sign of weakness or as a bid for attention. There are, also, gender differences, in that 'big boys don't cry', whereas women are allowed to cry in certain well-defined circumstances. Hence, when someone *does* cry, it becomes a cause for embarrassment.

A temptation is to comfort. 'Oh, please don't cry. Come on, why don't I make you a nice cup of tea? You will soon feel better.' Or, to cheer the individual up, 'Oh, surely not tears, look on the bright side. You have so much going for you. Come on, show me how brave you are.'

Either of the above strategies is likely to make the patient feel guilty; future grief may be contained, but the underlying cause of the grief will not be established, and feelings may be bottled up until a trigger explodes those feelings at a level which may require specialist help. If we take the case of a patient who is feeling insecure, she feels that her illness may alienate her partner, while he believes that she should trust to the strength of their feelings, without constant tangible reminders. He is too busy to shop for flowers on the way to the hospital, or to write letters on the days when he can't visit, and it simply doesn't occur to him that she will feel vulnerable and lonely. At visiting time it is she who conspires with the pretence, because their time is short and she does not wish him to be defensive or angry. As he leaves she manages to make her request, 'Write to me, darling', sound like a joke.

Sister, bringing the post, knows nothing of this. She sees a cancer patient who appears to have a concerned partner and lots of friends. Her disease is responding well to treatment. She will soon be back at work, and has everything to live for. Tears, then, are totally unexpected and unexplained. Contrast the following action with the words of comfort quoted earlier:

Sister:	You seem very upset. Let me get you a tissue.
Nan:	[Sniff] Sorry, Sister, you will think I'm stupid.
Sister:	[allowing time for the tears to stop] Please don't apologize.
Nan:	I don't often cry.
Sister:	Do you want to talk about it?
Nan:	Oh, you'll think I'm *so* stupid. In many ways I'm so lucky, but ...
Sister:	But ...?
Nan:	Well, it's knocked me, being in hospital like this ... and I really don't know how John feels. He says it makes no difference, but I'm not sure.
Sister:	Have you talked about it?
Nan:	How can I? He has never been one to talk about feelings. Even in the early days he teased me for being too analytical, and really, it hasn't mattered, because he is very loving most of the time.
Sister:	And now?
Nan:	Oh, I know it's me. I know he is busy and can't visit every day, but he works with a lot of women, younger than me, and I worry that he will turn to one of them. After all, they don't have my problems. I know it's silly, but if he would just put a card in the post or drop me a note, then I'd know he was thinking of me ... that I am important. Oh, Sister, I told you you would think I was stupid.
Sister:	No, Nan, not stupid. It's obviously very important to you. Tell me, is there any other reason for your distress?
Nan:	Well, not knowing about the future makes it worse.

In this interaction, Sister has gained a clear picture of the immediate distress and also factors which exacerbate it. Even though the tears have stopped, she has still to return to the cues about 'being knocked by the illness' and 'not knowing about the future' before she can help Nan decide how she is going to resolve the differing perceptions that she and John hold, or what other steps she might take to reduce her feelings of vulnerability.

To summarize, distress needs to be acknowledged and space must be given for the patient to regain control. After that, the opportunity should be given for the cause of the distress to be explored and clarified, before any intervention can be planned. In Nan's case, no advice was given on how to handle her partner; indeed, action plans were not suggested until all problems surrounding her distress were elicited. The important point is that if comfort alone had been offered, there would have been a real risk to the relationship as Nan became more insecure and John more impatient. In fact, the eruption, when it came, which would have been a distinct possibility, might well have taken the form of anger, not necessarily directed towards John, or related explicitly to Nan's hurt.

Anger may present as a difficulty for nurses and doctors, particularly when it seems illogical, unjustified, and inappropriately focused (Faulkner *et al.* 1994). The anger may be openly expressed or may present as a withdrawal from previously open interaction, with an attendant risk of eruption.

The angry patient
Inappropriate focus
Let us stay with Nan. Her concern has arisen owing to her stay in hospital and her belief that the constraints imposed by her illness will make her less attractive to John than one of the pretty girls with whom he works. She feels that she must not get angry with John for his lack of understanding, in case she drives him away. If a nurse has dealt with her distress by comfort alone, tears must be suppressed. One day the build-up of emotion erupts upon an unsuspecting nurse, as Nan says, 'I'm just a body in a bed to you. No one cares about me. I'm sick of it all. Oh. God, I can't stand much more of this.'

A common strategy when faced with this sort of outburst is to become defensive or go into battle, saying something like 'Of course we care. I know it's hard for you, but we are doing our best for you', or, 'That's naughty. You shouldn't say things like that. You are lucky compared to Mrs Smith over there.' What is more effective is to acknowledge the anger and try to defuse it by letting the patient ventilate her feelings. For example:

Nurse:	[in response to outburst] You sound very angry.
Nan:	Well, wouldn't you be, cooped up here? 'Take your tablets, dear ... Have a bath.' Oh God, where will it end?
Nurse:	Go on.
Nan:	Oh, I know they say I'm getting better; but they don't think. I've got a life to lead, and I don't know what's happening while I'm away.
Nurse:	What do you think might be happening?
Nan:	But that's it. No, it isn't your fault; but I'm so worried.
Nurse:	So worried?
Nan:	Yes, about John. He's with his mother while I'm in here, and she doesn't make an effort for him. I can't care for him or be with him. How can I expect him to go on loving me?

It will be seen that the patient's anger is defused; she has acknowledged that it was inappropriately focused, and has also disclosed her underlying worries, which had previously been suppressed. The nurse has accepted the patient's anger and stayed with it until the real cause of the hostility (anger about disease and hospitalization putting her relationship at risk) has been established, and the real problem of insecurity has been addressed.

Justified anger

Anger may be justified, for health professions *do* make mistakes, and occasionally make errors of judgement which, if the patient is aware, may rebound in terms of complaints and anger. The principles of dealing with justified anger are similar to those of dealing with *any* anger, i.e. acknowledgement, legitimizing (if appropriate), and exploration with the aim that the anger will be defused.

If anger takes the form of a verbal attack on a colleague, it is important not to rush to his/her defence. It may be that a patient is angry because he feels that the consultant has lied to him in view of subsequent events. A junior doctor may respond by saying, 'Oh, you must be wrong. He is a very good consultant.' This is only likely to exacerbate anger. A better approach is to explore the reasons for the belief that misinformation has been given, and then take appropriate action; not to take sides against a colleague, but to acknowledge that things do not always work out as we hope and that occasionally things do go wrong. It is interesting that, in general, people who go to litigation with their complaints are often those who have not been given the opportunity to explore their feelings with those who have upset them. In other words, genuine mistakes can be accepted if the reactions are explored in a caring manner, and justified anger acknowledged. It is important, where possible, to suggest that angry patients should take their anger to the person concerned, for no one should be expected to take responsibility for the actions of another.

Misdirected anger

Occasionally, anger may be expressed that is unjustified. A classic example is of the relative, worn out with caring for the loved one, who is encouraged to have a break by agreeing to respite care for the loved one. So often, the patient dies soon after admission to Hospice; and this event may be followed by an angry relative accusing the Hospice staff of neglect.

The first reaction may well be the desire to defend the care given; but this could lead to escalating anger. As before, it is necessary to acknowledge, diffuse, and explore the true focus of the anger. Consider the following exchange:

Mrs Black:	Ron was all right at home—I cared for him; you lot here have killed him—only 12 hours here and you let him die.
Doctor:	I can see that you are very angry and upset; but I do not believe that it all rests with us.
Mrs Black:	But he was fine at home.
Doctor:	Go on.
Mrs Black:	Well—not fine; but OK—I managed.
Doctor:	So?
Mrs Black:	Oh Doctor, I'd promised him he would die at home— I let him down. [starts crying]

In the above sequence, through encouraging Mrs Black to verbalize her feelings it became obvious that the outburst was more related to guilt than to anger. Such insight does not always come so readily; but is possible if people are encouraged to disclose their real feelings.

Pathological anger

Pathological anger is rare, and does not respond to the strategies used for justified and for inappropriately focused anger. In fact, if the individual were encouraged to express the anger, it could become violent. When faced with pathological anger, it is important to exert strong control to stop the outburst, and to refer on for specialist help.

In summary, anger may be justified, inappropriately focused, or pathological. All anger should be acknowledged, made legitimate if possible, explored, and defused. Only in pathological anger should firm control of the anger be exerted. It is worth noting here that some individuals have an angry approach to life in general. This should still be explored, in case there is legitimate cause for the outburst.

Difficult questions

Any individual, finding him- or herself in a new situation, tries to make sense of what is happening. Past experience may help, or knowledge gleaned from the media or family and friends; but eventually the picture may only become complete if certain central questions are answered. The questions that cancer patients often ask are difficult, in that they may address emotionally-loaded issues such as diagnosis, prognosis, and the efficacy of treatment. The difficulty may be compounded if there is not clear agreement within the team on how honest to be with any individual patient.

The situation may become more difficult when questions are indirect, because the doctor or nurse needs to explore cues to identify exactly what the patient is asking. Few patients, for example, ask the direct question, 'Am I going to die?' Rather they may say, 'Doesn't look too good, does it?' or 'My brother had this and he died' or, more directly, 'I can't see me getting over this, can you?' These and other similar statements are clear indications that the patient is thinking about death.

Questions about the diagnosis and treatment are equally difficult, since there is still a common belief that cancer equals death, and that cancer treatment causes more problems than it solves. In general, the effective way to deal with this sort of question is first to establish what exactly is being asked, and then why it is being asked, whether the patient really wants to know, and what is his or her current perception of the situation. What is not useful is premature or false reassurance, or a bid to make patients feel guilty about their apparent lack of trusting faith in their care. Compare the following responses to a patient with carcinoma of the liver:

A.

Joe:	How long will my skin be yellow?
Doctor:	It's just a touch of jaundice. Now, I've been talking to your wife. We thought you might be happier at St Columba's.
Joe:	Isn't that for cancer patients?
Doctor:	My, you are in the dumps today, and me trying to do my best for you.

B.

Joe:	How long will my skin be yellow?
Doctor:	What makes you ask that?
Joe:	Well, my old drinking buddy, Fred, went like this, feeling awful, skin yellow, and he died.
Doctor:	Go on.
Joe:	I guess I think I'm going to die too.
Doctor:	And how does that leave you feeling?
Joe:	I tell myself I've had a good life. I don't want to go, but in a funny way I know it's time.

This patient was looking for confirmation of what was happening to him. He gained this in the second interaction, where the doctor allowed him to explore his feelings; but he may still need to talk more. Any future discussion, however, will be based on Joe's reality rather than on the assumptions of professionals of what Joe *should* be told. This contrasts with the first interaction, where Joe is given clear signals that he will not have his questions answered.

One rationale for *not* answering difficult questions is that patients do not really want to know the answers. In fact, this can (and should) be clearly established since there is always a possibility that a question may be regretted as soon as it is asked. Had Joe, for example, been worrying about his yellow skin and fearful of the answer, his fear may have overcome his need for information, even though he asked the question—as follows:

Joe:	How long will my skin be yellow?
Doctor:	What makes you ask that?
Joe:	Oh, nothing really. My wife says I worry too much. I know I'm in good hands.

In the above exchange Joe is clearly backing off; but the doctor is alerted to the fact that Joe is beginning to think seriously of his prognosis, and may raise the subject again.

Nell Timms guessed she might be dying, so one day in November she said to the district nurse, 'I'll not make the clinic appointment in January, will I?'

The nurse deliberately missed the cue by replying 'Oh, I don't know. The roads may not be too bad', and then changed the subject. This nurse was unsure of how to proceed if the patient wanted a dialogue on her very uncertain prognosis, and needed time to gear herself to get into this very difficult area.

It is often argued that, in dealing with difficult questions, cues should be picked up as soon as they are given; but this is not necessarily true. Even experienced interviewers can miss cues, and cues which *are* picked up may be better dealt with at a later point in the interview, though once recognized cues should be acknowledged in a caring way, such as 'I can see that you are worried about that, and I *will* come back to it later, but first I'd like you to tell me a bit more about ...'. Most patients are happy with this, or will tell you if they are not.

Missed cues are not necessarily the disaster they are made out to be, since, when people have something on their minds, they will keep introducing the topic until it is noted, even if the reference is obscure. Nell Timms, for example, waited until the next time the district nurse visited her. While she was being bathed she said, 'They didn't save the King, did they, Nurse?' The nurse replied, 'No, I'm afraid not.' Nell was quiet for a while, and then said, 'So they won't save me.' In the ensuing conversation the nurse established that Nell knew that she had cancer (as had our last king) and that her prognosis was poor. She had wanted to 'bring the truth into the open' so that she could complete unfinished business and make her peace with a sister-in-law with whom she had had a silly quarrel.

One particular problem in dealing with difficult questions may be constraints imposed by consultants or relatives. Consultants may decide that it is in the patients' best interest to remain ignorant of diagnosis and prognosis, while relatives may wish to save them from the pain of knowledge. How health professionals can deal effectively with such collusion, while avoiding conflict, is discussed in Chapter 9 in regard to dealing with relatives, and Chapter 8 in relation to acting as the patient's advocate.

In summary, it can be seen that dealing with difficult questions should never degenerate into a 'to tell or not to tell' decision, but should be based on meeting the patient's expressed need for information. The prime objective in such a situation is carefully to establish the need for information and then to meet it in the light of the patient's current knowledge and perceptions.

Opting out of treatment

Occasionally, as patients' questions are answered, they may begin to question the sense of continuing treatment. They may believe that the short time left to them might be more pleasant without treatment, so allowing them to spend their remaining days at home with their families. Such thoughts may be in direct conflict with those of the health-care team, who may feel that a further course of treatment may 'buy time' for the patient which is worth the cost of side-effects.

A difficult situation may arise if the patient has unrealistic expectations of discontinuing treatment or if the medical team are over-zealous in prescribing at the expense of the patient's quality of life. If faced with a patient who wishes to opt out of treatment, the health professional should assess the situation to establish that the patient is, in fact, making an informed rather than a purely emotional choice. This is more effective, in terms of achieving the best possible option for any particular patient, than to use the strategy of claiming 'medical expertise' to diminish the patient's perspective and ensure compliance.

The following conversations show the two approaches used with a young patient suffering from leukaemia:

A.

Tessa:	I've been thinking about things, and I want to stop treatment and go home to get on with my life.
Doctor:	But you can't do that, Tessa. We have great hopes of this new treatment.
Tessa:	So you did about the last lot. It's time I faced reality.
Doctor:	The reality is that we have put a lot of investment into you—you can't let us down now.
Tessa:	That sounds like blackmail.
Doctor:	[affronted] Oh, no, we know what is best for you— and that is not allowing you to give up on your treatment.
Tessa:	But I must go home. I tell you, I've had enough.
Doctor:	Think of your family.
Tessa:	[angry] Just for once I'm thinking of me.
Doctor:	Well, I'm not going to argue with you. I've done my best.

B.

Tessa: I've been thinking about things, and I want to stop treatment and go home to get on with my life.

Doctor: Can you tell me why you want to do that, Tessa?

Tessa: Well, the last treatment didn't work, and I don't have much faith in this new one.

Doctor: It's difficult, because it's such early days yet, but we hope it will help you.

Tessa: But you aren't sure?

Doctor: No, though we are hopeful. It sounds as if the uncertainty is worrying you.

Tessa: Yes, because *I* hope—and I don't want to be disappointed again.

Doctor: So?

Tessa: So I know I won't get better, and if I stopped treatment I'd at least know where I stand. I could go home.

Doctor: I understand that—but you know, the treatment *might* give you more time. Would it help if you had some time at home and just came in briefly on treatment days?

Tessa: [thoughtfully] It might.

Doctor: Why don't you think it over and then we can talk again?

Tessa: OK. Yes, I'll do that.

In the first encounter, the doctor says that he has 'done his best', but in fact he has tried to change the patient's mind without attempting to understand her perspective. As a result the patient becomes stubborn and angry. In the second encounter, the doctor has tried to understand the patient's perspective and then offered alternatives to her 'all or nothing' approach to the problem. Because she is not under pressure, Tessa may well decide to complete the course of treatment.

Some patients, becoming doubtful about their treatment, may present a difficulty for the nurse or doctor by asking advice about alternative, or complementary, therapy. Again, the aim should be to help the patient to make an informed decision. This may be especially difficult if the health professional has strong views on complementary therapies, because personal bias made obvious may influence the patient's final decision.

The problem with giving definite advice on such a subject is that there is too little known about the effects for anyone to give knowledgeable advice. As a result, if patients decide *not* to try complementary therapy they may blame the nurse or doctor if they subsequently hear of someone who did well on it. Alternatively, if they do give up conventional treatment and go for complementary therapy, they may blame those who advised them if it does not succeed. This situation is less 'black and white' than formerly, since many patients continue conventional therapy *and* take up complementary options. The professional, in this difficult situation, needs to help patients make their own decisions on the basis of the available information. This requires assessment of patients to establish why they are considering complementary treatment, and then helping them to understand the implications so that their eventual choices are based in reality. This changes the role of the professional to that of a facilitator rather than an adviser, and carries the difficulty of seeing choices made which may conflict with professional beliefs.

In summary, when patients want to abandon treatment, or change to an alternative or complementary therapy, the professional should avoid rushing in with inappropriate advice, but rather, through assessment, give patients the information they need to make an informed choice.

Summary

In this chapter, a number of difficult situations have been considered, along with effective strategies for handling them. In no instance is this an easy task for the health professional, who may feel drained by the patient's emotions. Chapter 12 will deal with the resultant problems of the professional's survival. Not all difficult situations have been covered—some are dealt with elsewhere, such as euthanasia, and some may be unique to a certain area. It is hoped that the principles explained here will generalize to more specific problems.

References

Faulkner, A., Maguire, P., and Regnard, C. (1994). Dealing with anger in a patient or relative—a flow diagram. *Palliative Medicine*, **8**, 1, 51–7.

Maguire, P., Faulkner, A., and Regnard, C. (1993*a*). Handling the withdrawn patient—a flow diagram. *Palliative Medicine*, **8**, 76–81.

Maguire, P., Faulkner, A., and Regnard, C. (1993*b*). Managing the anxious patient with advanced disease—a flow diagram. *Palliative Medicine*, **7**, 239–44.

8

Handling conflict in cancer care

Introduction

The health professional will inevitably encounter situations in daily practice where the potential for interpersonal conflict is high. This chapter seeks to provide guidelines to help deal with these situations constructively. A common requirement is the willingness to confront individuals promptly once conflict arises, in a way that makes resolution reasonably likely. If health professionals are to be able to confront in this way they have to be willing to be assertive and represent their own views firmly, without alienating other people.

Patient advocacy

An experienced health professional may feel strongly that a patient or relative is not having the optimal treatment for his or her disease. This may be because the clinician responsible for key decisions about care is not fully aware of the situation, or has disregarded views that might have enabled him or her to make a more appropriate decision about treatment. It may also be because the patient is unable to make clear the problems encountered with the present regimen. The problem for the health professional is how to make a strong case for patients who cannot make it themselves, in a way which will avoid alienating the clinician but persuade him or her to take constructive action on the patient's behalf. It is all too easy for the agenda to become a win–lose battle between the health professional and the clinician, so that the patient is forgotten.

Nurse Foster: Can I have a word with you about Mrs Foulds?

Dr Miles: Can't you see I'm busy? The surgery is full of patients.

Nurse Foster: But I wouldn't be bothering you if I wasn't worried about her.

Dr Miles: But I saw her myself only a few days ago, and she seemed fine.

Nurse Foster:	Well, she isn't fine now; and that's what I wanted to talk to you about. I think she is depressed.
Dr Miles:	Depressed? I can't believe that. She seemed cheerful when I saw her. I have known her a long time. It's not like her to get depressed. She has been coping with her cancer very well.
Nurse Foster:	I agree, but I don't think she has been telling you the whole truth about how she feels.
Dr Miles:	She certainly has in the past; I can't see why she should change her attitude to me now.
Nurse Foster:	The fact is, she has.
Dr Miles:	I find that hard to believe.
Nurse Foster:	Well, I want you to do something about her depression.
Dr Miles:	But I don't agree she is depressed. So I don't see any need to see her sooner.

In the next example the nurse ensures that she checks that the doctor has sufficient time to deal with what is an urgent matter. She presents the facts professionally and objectively in such a way that the doctor cannot ignore them and has to take constructive action:

Dr Miles:	Hello, I gather you wanted to see me about Mrs Foulds because something urgent has happened.
Nurse Foster:	When I went to see her yesterday she wasn't at all well. She was very depressed.
Dr Miles:	What do you mean depressed? She certainly wasn't when I saw her last week. Indeed, she seemed cheerful.
Nurse Foster:	She said that since she realized her cancer had returned she had become so low that she did not want to go on living. She actually talked of attempting suicide by taking a massive overdose.
Dr Miles:	That staggers me, because she seemed to be coping so well with her cancer, even when it came back.
Nurse Foster:	Yes. But not now. She has other signs of depression. She is complaining of waking early in the morning and not being able to get back to sleep. She says that is the worst time of day, when she feels absolutely black and despairing. She says she gets no let up from this depression, and she can't think how she is going to get through the next few days without doing something.

Dr Miles: In that case I'd better see her as a matter of urgency. Would you like to come with me, and we can see her together?

Nurse Foster: Yes, I would, thank you.

The nurse had already alerted the doctor that the situation was urgent and had negotiated that he was prepared to discuss it. This allowed her to come to the point and describe the important fact that the patient was both depressed and suicidal. The doctor clearly had to take this seriously, particularly as the nurse followed on to indicate that she had clearly elicited other important signs and symptoms of a major depressive illness. The doctor, therefore, had no alternative but to respond and deal with the situation.

This way of advocating a patient's needs in a professional manner allows the nurse, who had not previously worked with this doctor, to gain credibility. After a period of time the mere fact that she was concerned about a patient would probably have become sufficient for him to take it seriously. Earning credibility in this way is also important when doctors are trying to encourage a nurse or other health professional to take a course of action. It is important that they represent the facts in such a professional, objective, and efficient manner, and also pay heed to how busy their colleagues are and negotiate both the time and the place for the discussion.

Confronting colleagues about undesirable behaviours

Such confrontation is necessary when a health professional is showing a pattern of behaviour which is seriously interfering with the proper management of patients and/or relatives. The health professional will need to confront the individual with this behaviour with the aim of allowing that person to acknowledge any problems and change to behaviours that are more constructive. In this example, a consultant is being confronted by a senior sister who has been concerned about his spending much less time with patients with a poor prognosis as against patients who are perceived to be likely to have a better outcome.

Dr Evans: You said you wanted to see me about something important?

Sister Benton: Yes, I have been very concerned about what has been happening to some of our patients in the last few weeks.

Dr Evans: What do you mean?

Sister Benton:	Some of them have been getting angry and bitter, because they feel they have been neglected.
Dr Evans:	What do you mean?
Sister Benton:	Well, you will remember Mrs Eccles, the lady we treated with chemotherapy for cancer of the ovary.
Dr Evans:	Yes. I wasn't aware there was anything amiss.
Sister Benton:	Well, she knew that her disease had come back and that there hadn't been much of a response to chemotherapy. She was extremely worried about it, and wanted to talk to you about it. However, she said you only spent a minute or two with her, and then went off to see somebody else. She felt abandoned.
Dr Evans:	But I was only trying to do my best for her. I didn't think it would help to dwell on the fact that she had a very poor prognosis, particularly as she has such a young family.
Sister Benton:	I can understand that. But I think this has become part of a pattern. She is only one example of people you have tended to spend very little time with. We have had at least ten such patients in the last six months who feel they have been abandoned by you once things didn't seem to be working out.

As the interaction continued, Dr Evans moved from being defensive about his actions to admitting that he found the area increasingly hard to deal with. His sister had died of cancer in the last year, and he had obviously some unresolved grief which made him feel vulnerable when faced with others who were coming to grips with a poor prognosis.

By being confronted with the reality of the situation in a manner that he could acknowledge and accept, Dr Evans gained insight into his current problems and their effect on his work and interactions with dying patients. This allowed Dr Evans to admit that because of a very bad personal experience in his family he had found it hard to stay with patients whose cancer had a poor prognosis.

It is helpful to regard this confronting of colleagues as equivalent to breaking bad news. It should be made clear to the individual at the outset that the topic of the discussion is a serious one. Time should not be spent in small talk, otherwise this will give a wrong connotation to the interview. The individual will then be more likely to become angry when the confrontation occurs. It is also important to have solid evidence about the undesirable behaviours and their consequences to present to the people being confronted, so that they cannot use alibis to sidestep the complaints. Only then is it likely that they will acknowledge that there is a problem.

Sister Benton negotiated whether or not she could explore underlying reasons for Dr Evans' behaviour. Some individuals may be unwilling to share this more personal information, and yet may still be willing to consider changing their policies or behaviours.

Commonly, such confrontations are left until too many strong feelings have developed within a team. It is then hard to confront the issue with-out its becoming a 'battleground', and an issue of win or lose. As with patient advocacy, the key is to keep the importance of the patients and relatives at the centre of the discussion, along with concern for the colleague and his or her current problems.

Far too often, health professionals argue that the individuals concerned are incapable of changing. However, the greater problem is usually the reluctance to give them the kind of feedback that would promote change. Individuals who are alleged to be incapable of change can often change greatly if they are provided with the necessary information in the right manner, and understanding is shown of their particular difficulties.

It can also help, as long as it is true, to indicate that the undesirable behaviours represent a change from what had previously been a good working relationship. Thus, Sister Benton might have said 'I am concerned because your reluctance to spend much time with these patients represents a great change from what you used to do a year or so ago, when we seemed to have very few problems with your patients. Then they were all very satisfied with the care they were getting.'

When the undesirable behaviour is such that it is seriously interfering with colleagues' ability to work, yet the individual at fault has no insight or refuses to change, the issue may have to become a disciplinary matter between the appropriate health professionals. Moreover, the health professional may have to explain that he or she has to appeal to someone at a higher level.

Conflict with patients
While colleagues can provoke conflict, patients may also cause problems for the health professional for a number of reasons.

The demanding patient
Even when a counselling relationship has been contracted properly and the number and duration of the sessions negotiated and agreed, there are

patients who will still try to demand more time than is justified. Even in a one-off assessment interview the patient may demand a lot more time than is available. Here, it is important to set limits, to educate the patient about what is possible, and to be prepared to renegotiate for further appointments if necessary.

Dr Purvis: I am afraid our time is nearly up.

Mrs Seaton: Oh, it can't be, I have only been here a few minutes.

Dr Purvis: I am afraid it is. We have had our forty minutes. I would just like to recap what we have discussed in this session.

Mrs Seaton: It's simply not good enough.

Dr Purvis: I am not prepared to extend the sessions, because this is the time we negotiated and agreed was appropriate to the problems you wanted help with. If you feel you need more help than this we can explore that next time, and establish in what way you feel I am not helping you sufficiently. Maybe we could begin the next session doing that.

Mrs Seaton: You are just no bloody good at all, are you?

Dr Purvis: I am simply making it clear that this is the basis on which we agreed to work. If you can accept that then I would be happy to see you again and discuss it.

It is all too easy to be blackmailed into spending more time with a given patient. Other patients booked into a clinic or who are to be visited at home then inevitably get less time as the day goes on. Alternatively, the health professional works over-long hours and is thus at risk of becoming increasingly drained and less effective. It is very important to negotiate time with patients, and to expect co-operation from them. Most patients appreciate time constraints and know when they can expect to leave after an appointment.

Mrs Seaton's demand was blatant and the response firm. It is more difficult when demands are more subtle, but it is important to deal with them sooner rather than later. Pressure to befriend a patient or relative can present particular problems.

Mrs Adams: I have felt increasingly lonely because the family are out all day. I just wish I had someone to talk with. I find you easy to talk with, very easy.

Nurse Connors: Would you like me to come round occasionally and talk to you then?

Mrs Adams: Yes, I would like that very much.

Here the specialist nurse had fallen into the trap of offering time which could well have been filled by the patient's other relatives or friends. She should have encouraged the patient to make the effort to do that rather than seek to fill the void herself, and become more of a friend than a professional worker.

The situation could have been handled like this:

Mrs Adams: I have felt increasingly lonely because the family are out all day. I just wish I had someone to talk with. I find you easy to talk with, very easy.

Nurse Connors: Thank you. Who else do you know that you get on well with, and who might be willing to come and see you from time to time and try to help you with the loneliness? It is hard when you have to stay in the house.

Mrs Adams: Do you think they would come?

Nurse Connors: Well, give it some thought, and then perhaps you could phone a friend and see if she would like to drop by.

In the above exchange, Mrs Adams is encouraged to take some action to contact friends and arrange a meeting.

Nurse Connors' aim is to empower the patient to resolve the problem rather than to do it for her; and she can then monitor progress. The request to befriend can be very seductive; but it is important to resist it, since it blurs professional boundaries. It also leads patients and relatives to have unrealistic expectations of what the health professional might be able to deliver, and may cause problems within a family. For example, the patient or relative may turn increasingly to the health professional as a source of support rather than to a partner or close relative.

Befriending can be a particular danger when trying to help somebody recently bereaved (Chapter 11). Here, the bereaved person may be tempted to fill the gap in his or her life by leaning increasingly on the health professional. This can create an unhelpful dependency and make it difficult for the health professional to sever the relationship.

Transference

A transference is said to arise when the patient begins to develop feelings for the health professional as though that health professional represented an important person in the patient's past or present life. These feelings are 'unconscious', so that the patient is not aware of the basis of them.

The transference may take a dependent form, where patients begin to feel that the health professional is going to meet all their needs to the extent that the other person did in earlier life. When the health professional fails to meet the needs to this extent patients can become extremely angry. Alternatively, patients may have felt abandoned in earlier life because a parent died or parents divorced. The health professional may then find that simple behaviours, like being slightly late for an appointment, lead to the patient becoming unreasonably angry. Confronting the patient with her anger and inviting her to consider possible reasons will usually reveal that she is terrified of being abandoned. Inviting the patient to further consider whether she had ever felt abandoned like this in the past will usually allow her to make the connection with the original abandonment that has led to this fear.

Some patients may become extremely upset when they feel that they are being criticized by the health professional within an interview. The health professional should be aware that such sensitivity is not an objective reaction to how he or she is behaving, but represents an over-sensitivity on the part of the patient. Acknowledgement of this apparent over-sensitivity and negotiation to explore the reasons will usually reveal that the patient has experienced harsh criticism in the past, usually from a parent or close relative.

When individuals have experienced sexual abuse in early life they may begin to fear that the therapist will actually attack them at some stage during the therapeutic relationship. Thus they may move their chair back suddenly and look very frightened, particularly if the therapist has made some physical movement towards them.

For these reasons it is important to be aware of signs of transference. When an inappropriate behaviour begins to emerge on the part of the patient it is important to consider whether a transference might have developed, and to explore this possibility:

Nurse Timms: Over the last few sessions you seem to have been getting increasingly irritated with me. Whenever I make a comment you seem to take it as a criticism, and seem hurt and angry. Is that at all possible?

Miss Clark: Yes, I have been getting really pissed off with you.

Nurse Timms: Can you say why that is?

Miss Clark: I feel you are getting more critical of me. I feel you don't really respect me as a person.

Nurse Timms: I am a bit puzzled by that, because I don't honestly think my behaviour and attitude towards you has

	changed. Could it be that in some way I remind you of somebody from the past who was very critical of you?
Miss Clark:	Yes: you are just like my mother.
Nurse Timms:	Can you bear to say in what way?
Miss Clark:	Well, for one thing you look like her, you are the same kind of age, and you have the same kind of authoritarian attitude.
Nurse Timms:	No wonder, then, that you have been feeling criticized and got at. Perhaps we could explore that a bit more?
Miss Clark:	Yes, OK.

The important thing here is that the nurse counsellor has sufficient personal awareness and insight to know that she was not being critical or insensitive. She also realized the importance of checking out whether a transference had developed, and found out she was related to as though she were the patient's mother, who had indeed been over-critical and insensitive during the patient's childhood and adolescence. She still found her mother difficult to relate to.

A transference reaction can also take a positive form, in which the patient begins to feel very positively about the health professional as a person. Patients may begin to idealize health professionals, and look to them to solve problems when no solutions may be possible. They may actually come to love the health professional, and this may take a sexual form, in which the patient fantasizes having a sexual relationship with the health professional. It is especially important to be vigilant to such positive transference. Early signs are patients turning up very early for appointments, taking particular care to look attractive, trying to make contact between sessions, and making positive personal comments about the health professional during sessions or by means of letters.

Conflict may also arise when the health professional develops a counter-transference to the patient. Here the patient reminds the health professional of someone she disliked or was very fond of in her own personal life. This can create tension and turmoil unless the health professional realizes what is happening by introspecting about why that patient is making her feel uncomfortable or why she is making extra-special efforts to help this patient, and getting over-involved. If such introspection fails to reveal any useful answers it is worth discussing the situation with a supervisor.

If the health professional discovers that she is repeatedly experiencing certain patients as difficult to work with because she gets over-involved or angry too easily she needs to discuss this with an appropriate supervisor. The supervisor may be able to help her identify the basis of the difficulty and help her resolve it. Alternatively, she may discern that the difficulties are too substantial to be resolved easily, and advise the health professional to seek more expert advice.

When a specific situation consistently triggers the health professional it is sensible to advise her to avoid taking on that kind of individual, and to request colleagues to do so.

Role conflict

Strong feelings of conflict may be provoked when there is uncertainty about the precise role that individuals play within a team when trying to help patients with cancer and their relatives. Individuals can feel extremely threatened if they perceive that another health professional is seeking to take over the same territory. It is important to confront this situation early and to try and resolve it to mutual benefit.

Father Peters: Thank you for coming to talk to me. I think it very important that we discuss our respective roles in terms of the spiritual care of patients in the hospice.

Sister Richards: I can't understand what the problem is. We are perfectly able to advise patients about their spiritual problems. Of course if we get out of our depth we call you in.

Father Peters: But that's the problem. At the moment I only seem to be called in rarely. I am certain there are more patients that could benefit from my help than I am seeing.

Sister Richards: What makes you think that?

Father Peters: Well, I've had to talk to people shortly before their death on several occasions recently. On each occasion I found they had concerns that simply hadn't been dealt with by anybody.

Sister Richards: Can you give me an example?

Father Peters: Yes, I can give you several. Would you like me to?

Sister Richards: I need convincing.

Father Peters was then able to illustrate very clearly the ways in which some patients were not getting the spiritual help and guidance they needed. He went on to discuss with Sister Richards those indications that should suggest to a nurse that a chaplain like himself should be called in to help.

Sister Richards, albeit reluctantly, agreed to consider this and give it a try. Such role conflict is usually the result of a sense of insecurity on the part of one of the professionals. Open discussion and negotiation are then required in order to improve trust in the working relationship.

Summary

However well health professionals communicate with cancer patients and relatives they will inevitably encounter conflicts of various sorts. These conflicts are usually resolvable provided they are approached constructively and the health professional has a reasonable degree of personal awareness. Having a good knowledge of professional versus personal boundaries can prevent many of the conflicts arising.

9

Talking to relatives

In previous chapters, the emphasis has been on identifying the patients' problems and encouraging them to generate possible solutions. It is too easy to forget that relatives may also have problems in coping with a loved one's illness, and may need professional help, especially as they often feel that they are not entitled to disclose problems because the patient is seen to be the priority.

Patients and relatives may have differing perspectives about their predicament and have competing needs. The illness may throw relationships out of balance, for relatives often take on the task of making decisions about what is best for their loved ones. This can lead to collusion, disagreements about who should be told what, and other related problems.

The health professional needs to be able to identify family problems and to identify those problems connected to the cancer situation, as opposed to those that are long-standing. The latter are unlikely to be solved because one family member has cancer, but can cause problems for carers who may not understand the consequent tensions.

Family dynamics
Family dynamics are important, particularly if the family is large, or has conflicting interests or an overbearing family member who may wish to 'take control' at the expense of others.

Family spokesperson
A common problem, where there are several close family members, is that they may all claim equal rights to information and make regular telephone calls asking for information that is already in the possession of one relative. The arguments can be quite powerful, for example:

Nurse: [answering telephone] Hello, this is Ward 8.
Mr Mollington: Hello, I'm Joe Mollington. Can you tell me the situation with my mother?

Nurse:	Well, the doctor spoke to your father today. Your mother is comfortable.
Mr Mollington:	I would like more information than her comfort.
Nurse:	I suggest you talk to your father.

The above situation leaves the relative feeling that he is being blocked, while the nurse is left feeling that she has better things to do than give the same information to several members of the family.

Such difficulties can be avoided by asking the patient to take responsibility for nominating the person who should be the family spokesperson. If the patient is too ill, this responsibility rests with the next of kin. It should be explained that by nominating one person, unnecessary problems can be avoided.

Nurse:	[at end of assessment interview] Well, Mrs Mollington, we hope you will be comfortable with us. I know that your family are very concerned about you, but to make sure we get things right, I'd like you to tell me who we should contact if the need arises, and who we should give information to. It's usually best to have just one person, and he or she will know who needs to be told of your progress.
Mrs Mollington:	Oh! Well, it had better be Ted, my husband—the boys quarrel among themselves, but Ted keeps them straight, and he will tell them what we decide they need to know; and my daughter, well, she's going through divorce at the moment—she doesn't need any more on her plate.
Nurse:	Fine; well, let's leave it at that for now, and see how we go.

In the above exchange, the patient is left feeling in control of the situation, and the nurse has a clear picture of how to proceed with the family.

The dominant relative

Clear understanding between health professional and key family members does not necessarily solve all problems. Many families have a dominant relative, who may try to bully staff to gain information. However, if a clear agreement exists on who is the family spokesperson, the health professional can be assertive.

Mr Shelbourne:	I'm needing some information about my sister, Mrs Mollington. How is she—what's her outlook—should I come to see her?
Registrar:	Mrs Mollington is very comfortable, and has been up in the dayroom today. I suggest you have a word with her husband about visiting.
Mr Shelbourne:	Comfortable! That's what you all say.
Registrar:	Well, we agreed with Mrs Mollington and her husband that he is our link person. We find that we avoid tensions by having one family spokesperson. Then it is up to the patient and that person to liaise with the rest of the family.
Mr Shelbourne:	Ted! Let me tell you that I've had to get my sister out of many a scrape with Ted.
Registrar:	Mr Shelbourne, I'm afraid I cannot get involved in family conflicts. I'll tell Mrs Mollington that you telephoned and are concerned about her.

The Registrar was pleasant but firm, because there were clear guidelines on the giving of information about the patient's diagnosis and prognosis.

The lonely relative

Although large families present the potential for problems, there is also an inherent problem if the patient has only one or two close relatives. This is more likely if the patient is elderly and his or her partner or relative is frail. It is important to elicit what other support, if any, is available, such as a neighbour, so that if bad news has to be broken there is someone available to offer help and be present if necessary.

For individuals who are alone and have no support, a community nurse or a member of the clergy should be available if bad news has to be given.

The outcast

It is not unusual for families with long-standing feuds to exclude a family member from involvement. The 'outcast' may find out, by chance, that a relative has cancer and is very ill. If no arrangement has been made for a family spokesperson, health professionals may find that they are criticized for giving information to the 'outcast' or allowing him or her access to the patient.

One of Mrs Mollington's sons, David, had moved in with his Indian girlfriend, to the horror of his family. He heard by chance that his mother was ill and visited her at lunchtime one day.

Before the split, David and his mother had been very close. She was pleased to make her peace with him. He visited at times when no one else came, until his father arrived as he was leaving one day.

Mr Mollington went to the ward sister's office and complained about his son's being allowed in. The sister asserted that this was a matter between the couple and their son. Mrs Mollington admitted that she had encouraged David, and a truce was agreed, although David and his father remained cool with each other.

It is more difficult when the 'outcast' is a mistress or a homosexual lover who is not acceptable to the family, but who loves and is concerned for the patient. Here, the responsibility rests with the patient and the person concerned. It is not the responsibility of the health professional to take on these problems.

Interacting effectively with family members can enhance the comfort of the patient and his relatives, and allow other problems to be dealt with as they arise.

Collusion

One major difficulty for relatives may be in facing the serious diagnosis and prognosis of a loved one. This can become apparent through denial or over-optimism; but a classic reaction is to request health professionals to collude in protecting the patient from the truth. If the doctor shares the diagnosis and outlook with the relative *before* talking to the patient, the relative is often able to make a strong case for collusion, which is difficult for the health professional to dispute.

Jane Brown's husband was told that her cancer had not responded to treatment. Although Mrs Brown was feeling fairly hopeless about her future, she put on a brave face for Harry, her husband. He argued that it was better for her to be encouraged to think positively, and asked the doctor not to tell her the truth. The doctor felt that Jane was ready for the truth, and tried to persuade Harry to change his mind.

Doctor: Mr Brown, I think it would be best if we were more honest with your wife.

Mr Brown: Look, I know Jane. She has always relied on me to protect her. She couldn't take the truth. She would just curl up.

Doctor: But she has to face reality one day.

Mr Brown:	[shouting] No! You mustn't hurt her like that. I won't have it—do you hear?
Doctor:	[sounding tired] Very well, but we may have to discuss this again.
Mr Brown:	And my answer will be the same.

The doctor did not succeed with Mr Brown because he did not understand the reasons for Mr Brown's apparent stubbornness. Careful assessment needs to be made to establish the relative's reasons for colluding. This should then allow the professional to negotiate a more open approach.

Such an assessment should concentrate first on the relative's perceptions and feelings about the current situation. It is commonly believed that relatives need collusion to protect *themselves* from pain, but usually the opposite is true. Collusion is more usually an act of love and a wish to protect a loved one from anguish. Mr Brown, for example, was not wanting comfort for himself. He loved his wife so much that he wished to save her from pain. Further, he truly believed that Jane would not be able to cope with her reality, and wanted to protect her as he had always been able to do in the past.

It is therefore important to elicit the relatives' perceptions of the illness to check that they themselves understand the true situation and are not in denial. After this, it is important to establish the *cost* of collusion.

Doctor:	Clearly, Mr Brown, you understand the seriousness of the situation, but tell me—how does that leave you feeling?
Mr Brown:	Well, I manage to keep a brave face. I have to for Jane, but sometimes ...
Doctor:	Sometimes ...?
Mr Brown:	Well, at night ... I wake up. Last week was her birthday, and I thought, would this be the last time? Silly really, she loves surprises, and I love to plan them. She had asked me not to buy a present this year till she was better, but I bought her a silly toy, a koala bear, but then I lay awake after I'd bought it, knowing I'd never be able to make her dream come true of a trip to Australia. I cried ... me, a grown man.
Doctor:	And is it often like that?
Mr Brown:	At night, yes. I think of all our plans and how they won't come true, and I worry that she doesn't really understand how much I love her.

Doctor:	Do you tell her?
Mr Brown:	I'm not that sort of man. I don't discuss feelings easily. She has always wanted to, but if I start now ... even if I could ... she would suspect.
Doctor:	And you think she doesn't?
Mr Brown:	Oh no, and I don't think she should know.
Doctor:	I'd like to come back to that, but first I want to check with you if you have other difficulties in keeping the truth from your wife?

In the above sequence, Mr Brown began to divulge the cost of collusion to him personally and in terms of emotional strain and the pressure on the relationship. The doctor was not diverted by Mr Brown's assertion that Jane should not be told, but remained with Mr Brown's concerns. What emerged was that Mr Brown felt isolated, did not sleep well, could no longer talk freely to Jane, and was finding difficulty in concentration when he was at work.

Only when the emotional cost of collusion and impact on the relationship have been identified should the matter of breaking collusion be raised. Even then it should not be presented as a challenge, nor as a moral obligation. We saw the effect of challenge earlier in this chapter. Compare that with the following interaction.

Doctor:	I can see that the cost of protecting Jane has been very high for you, Mr Brown.
Mr Brown:	But I'll willingly bear it for her.
Doctor:	I'm sure you will ... but tell me ... have you ever thought, even fleetingly, that she may know herself?
Mr Brown:	Well, that business over her birthday ... but ... no ...
Doctor:	Go on.
Mr Brown:	Well, she loves presents. I wondered ... her saying not to buy anything ... if she knew that she hasn't long.
Doctor:	I suspect that she might guess. I wonder if you would let me talk to her ... for if you both know, then it could be brought into the open, and it could make things easier for both of you.
Mr Brown:	If you mean, can you tell her, the answer is no. I know Jane. She has always relied on me to protect her. She couldn't take the truth ... she would just curl up.
Doctor:	I accept that you know Jane better than I do, and I can promise you that I won't just tell her that she is going to die. I would like to talk to her, and if, as we both suspect, she *does* know, then I would confirm it.

Mr Brown:	Is that a promise? You won't force her to face the truth?
Doctor:	Definitely not. If she really has no idea, then I'll just leave it. Could you be happy with that?
Mr Brown:	Yes, I can't have her hurt, but if she *does* know, then we could talk. It's so 'forced' between us at the moment.

Having gained permission for a dialogue, the health professional needs to assess the patient's awareness of the situation. If the patient is coping by denial, the collusion may have to stand. More often, however, the patient has not confided in her partner for the same reason as the relative has not given her the truth—because she loves him and wants to protect him. Also, she may have come to the conclusion that her time is limited, and she has not wanted the reality confirmed.

The health professional then may have the task of confirming prognosis in addition to divulging the fact that the partner is aware of the situation. This *may* cause repercussions, not least an angry response—in a patient who felt that hers was an honest open relationship beforehand. Either partner may feel unable to open the dialogue in which each accepts his or her part in the collusion. It may require the health professional to offer to bring the couple together and to concentrate on the positive emotions which allowed such a situation to arise. This 'presence' may only need to be brief for some couples—the situation will be highly charged; but for others they may need someone there to whom they can turn for help and advice.

Knowing how long to stay requires great sensitivity, as does knowing when to stay silent. It is possible to negotiate with the couple when the boundaries do not seem clear.

Jane:	You knew all along? Why didn't you say so?
Harry:	Darling, I wanted to save you from knowing.
Jane:	You could have trusted me enough to say *something*.
Doctor:	Shall I leave you? I feel you have private things to say.
Jane:	Don't go, it's all such a shock. Harry, darling, you have been so distant. I thought you didn't care. And me, I don't know what to expect.
Doctor:	We can talk about that later, but now I think I *should* leave you together.

Later, either or both partners may need to consult a health professional; but immediately the truth is in the open, this couple, as so many others, need to regain the emotional ground lost during collusion before all else, and may do this best alone without the constraints of a third party.

In summary, collusion usually happens because of a need to protect a beloved person from a painful truth. It is not an easy option for the colluder, and often carries a high emotional cost. The health professional's concern should be to promote a more open approach while maintaining the trust of those involved. A promise can always be made that information will only be given if the partner is ready to accept the truth. This promise, often seen as a constraint on the health professional, is in fact the key to breaking collusion, since, in making the promise, the health professional is respecting the knowledge and beliefs of the colluder while maintaining the right to answer questions and confirm the suspicions of the other person involved.

The health professional as agent of collusion
It used to be common for the doctor to make the decision to 'to tell' or 'not to tell'. This may still arise when a health professional believes it is best to withhold the truth from a patient. The reasons for this usually stem from the concept of 'a strong health professional protecting a weak patient'. The nurse may find herself thrown into the role of patient's advocate if it is the doctor's decision to collude; but too often little thought is given to the potential effect on the relatives, who are faced with a decision which may be difficult to accept.

That many relatives welcome the advice that the patient should not be told is undisputed. However, thought needs to be given to those relatives who function on a more honest basis. Fred and Mabel Black, for example, felt that their marriage was based on honesty and openness. When Mabel's leg began to swell and abdominal pain interfered with her day-to-day functioning, she asked Fred to be honest with her in terms of what the doctors said to him. Because she had nursed her mother in her final illness she had little faith that the doctors would be open with her.

The team in charge of Mabel's case decided it was best that she should *not* be told that she had ovarian carcinoma with metastases, but that she had 'internal pressures', which needed to be relieved by treatment.

Fred and the doctor found themselves in the reverse of Mr Brown's situation, since Fred felt that Mabel would want to know. The doctor was adamant:

Mr Black: Look doctor, my wife is no fool.

Doctor:	I'm sure she isn't; but the team don't believe she can take this news. It's my professional duty to protect her, and if you love her you will agree.
Mr Black:	But we are always open with each other!
Doctor:	But you haven't had such serious information before. Believe me, Mr Black, I know best.

Fred felt defeated by the doctor's arguments and went along with the collusion without a belief in its necessity. This subsequently caused difficulties with Mabel, who finally discovered the truth and blamed Fred for lack of loyalty and care.

Consider an alternative approach, with the same doctor respecting Fred's knowledge of his wife.

Mr Black:	Look doctor, my wife is no fool.
Doctor:	It sounds as if you don't agree that we should keep the truth from her.
Mr Black:	No, I don't. I watched Mabel when her mother was dying. She couldn't understand the doctor talking to her as the relative rather than Mum who was going through it all. She made me promise it wouldn't happen to her.
Doctor:	But your wife's situation is very grave.
Mr Black:	Yes, and I think she suspects that.
Doctor:	Would you like me to talk with her—assess where she is in terms of her illness?
Mr Black:	If you would; but then you wouldn't lie to her, would you?

In this latter example, both the doctor and Fred are agreeing a strategy to meet Mabel's need for knowledge at a level that she can handle. In the event, the doctor's role was to confirm Mabel's beliefs about the situation, after which *she* initiated an honest discussion with Fred.

Collusion occurs because an individual, for the best of motives, believes that he or she has a right or duty to withhold information from another person. This throws into sharp relief the whole question of whose information it is, how decisions are made about sharing information, and who should be giving such information.

Information

Giving information to the patient was discussed in Chapter 5. A common problem in giving information to relatives is whether it is best to talk to the patient and relative together or separately. At first sight this may appear a comparatively simple matter, in that all one needs to do is to ask the couple how they feel. There are, in fact, several problems inherent in this approach.

Dominant partner

Even in the most loving relationship, it is very likely that one partner will be more dominant than the other. How couples deal with this may differ if they are in public rather than in private. The dominant partner may 'take over' in an interaction with the doctor or nurse and not be challenged, as might be the case if they were having a difference of opinion in private.

Talking to such a couple together may well give a 'skewed' picture of their needs, for example:

Doctor:	Well, Mr and Mrs Hall, I felt it was time for us to review the situation. Would you like me to talk to you together?
John:	Yes, that would be the best idea.
Nan:	Don't you think …
John:	Look doctor, you won't want to say the same things twice. We'll talk to you together, won't we Nan?
Nan:	[quietly] Yes … yes, that's OK.
Doctor:	Are you sure, Mrs Hall?
Nan:	John is usually right, doctor. What did you want to talk about?

Nan's real feelings might have been elicited if the doctor had explored further with her; but asking the couple together caused difficulties for Nan. Her need to talk alone had to compete with her feelings of loyalty for her partner.

Whose information?

The above example raises the issue of whose information it is that is being discussed. Partners and relatives may feel that they are so involved in their loved one's life that they have equal rights to information. The reality is that doctors often share news with relatives *before* they do with the patient, especially when a diagnosis is serious or fear-provoking. This may be avoided by seeing a couple together initially, but could lead to a very difficult interview if the patient is not ready to share, or needs time to adapt before having a discussion with a partner.

Inhibitions

It may be that the presence of a partner will inhibit disclosure from a relative. This is particularly true where bad news is concerned (see Chapter 5), and one partner wants to present a more cheerful picture to the other; but may be equally true at any level of disclosure. It could be predicted, for example, that Nan Hall will be far less disclosing in the presence of John, so that her information needs will not get stated:

Doctor: Sister tells me that you were asking her questions about how things are going.

Nan: [hesitantly] Oh, I'm not really worried.

Doctor: Are you sure?

In fact, Nan *did* want an update on prognosis, but not in front of John, because she wanted to choose what was discussed with him. John put the final seal on the interaction by stepping in and reiterating that she was satisfied with the current level of information.

Inhibitions can seriously affect the exchange of information when there are problems in a relationship. These are not always apparent, since individuals tend to wear a 'public face' when together. It is unlikely, for example, for a wife to disclose in front of her husband that he beats her, keeps her short of money, or is not supportive.

If any of these things are true, however, the individual may need information on sources of help because she feels unable to cope alone. She may have to forfeit that help if her partner is present in an interview, simply because she dare not disclose the true nature of the problems.

Differential coping

Couples do not always cope in the same way with their day-to-day problems. Some may need to talk through their concerns with their partner. They would argue that this brings things into the open, clears the air, and allows joint decisions to be made on how to deal with a problem or reach a working compromise. Others are most uncomfortable with the notion of talking about any potentially painful situation, and get tense and angry if the topic is raised. Such people prefer to leave the subject alone and may say things such as, 'There is no point in discussion—it's unlikely to change the outcome' or 'Talking about it will just make it worse—the whole thing will blow up.'

Trying to give information to a couple when each has a different method of coping is likely to lead to hostility. One partner may need to talk about her cancer all the time, and will feel frustrated and hurt by her partner's silence. Surely if he loved her, her partner would accept her need to verbalize. He, on the other hand, can't bear to mention the cancer, but may be equally upset, thinking that she should know better than to try to raise issues, especially in front of the nurse or doctor. The doctor may well feel like a 'pig-in-the-middle'.

The need to negotiate

There are many factors to be considered before a decision is made on whether to involve relatives in the giving of information to a patient or to see the patient alone. Because it is not easy to pick up where a relationship 'is at' in terms of dominance, potential inhibitions, its strength, and each individual's coping mechanisms, negotiation should occur with each partner separately wherever possible. This may well result in the decision to be seen together; but hopefully each partner will have made the choice independently. It may, however, result in a decision on the patient's part *not* to have a partner present or for a partner to prefer not to be involved when a patient receives information about disease and its treatment.

These individual preferences should be respected as far as is possible, but may cause problems for the health professional if the couple's needs do not match. This is more likely to happen in the home or in the outpatients' department, where relatives can be quite insistent that they should stay with the patient and hear everything that is said.

In most cases, negotiation will work, particularly if the relative's need is acknowledged. What is to be avoided is a battle, for example:

District Nurse:	Hello, Mr Mottram. I've come to see your wife.
Mr Mottram:	She's upstairs. I'll come with you.
District Nurse:	I'd rather see her alone.
Mr Mottram:	I'd rather you didn't.
District Nurse:	Oh, surely; and anyway, I want to examine her.
Mr Mottram:	You won't see anything I haven't seen.
District Nurse:	I'm asking you to let me see her alone.
Mr Mottram:	And I'm telling you, NO. It's *my* house, *my* wife; and I'll not have a chit like you ordering us about.

What will undoubtedly work better is for the nurse to concentrate on Mr Mottram's concerns, as in collusion, and then negotiate for time.

In considering the involvement of a relative in any aspect of patient care, one has to accept that occasionally it will not be possible to get co-operation because of intractable belief or profound stubbornness. Such cases are rare, and if a skilled approach is used there is no need to feel a failure. It is more productive to concede that, having done your best, you still cannot expect to 'win them all'. Also, it should be remembered that assessment of relatives' problems, as is true for patients, is an ongoing activity, and as situations change, so may reactions. For example, while Mr Mottram didn't want his wife to know the truth, he protected her by his presence. Once collusion was broken, the situation was freed up, and he came to trust the nurse sufficiently that she was able to see his wife alone.

Treatment

Occasionally a relative may wish to be involved in treatment decisions, independently of the patient. It may be that a decision has been made to give no further treatment. A further course of chemotherapy may have been an option that the team believes to have little value in a patient with advanced disease and a very poor outlook. The patient may have accepted this news with relief; but his partner may try to insist that the extra course should be given.

In such situations, the response from the health professional may be defensive, or logical, or both, for example:

Mrs Lovatt: So you have abandoned him doctor? I think it is disgraceful!

Doctor: If you mean the treatment, I'm afraid it is pointless to give more, given the spread of the disease.

Mrs Lovatt: But another course may make all the difference.

Doctor: Let me explain ...

In the above sequence it is unlikely that the doctor will convince the relative. What is more likely to succeed is an attempt to understand the relative's concern:

Mrs Lovatt: So you have abandoned him doctor? I think it is disgraceful!

Doctor: I can see that you are upset—can you try to explain?

Mrs Lovatt: I want him to have more chemotherapy—and you are saying he can't. How can you justify that?

Doctor: I will tell you; but first I wonder why you are so keen for Leon to have more?

Mrs Lovatt: [long pause] Nothing has worked up to now ... but ...

Doctor: But?

Mrs Lovatt: Well, while he was on treatment, I had hope ...

Doctor: And now?

Mrs Lovatt: And now I have to accept ... Oh God! ... [starts crying]

In the above sequence the doctor has explored the relative's concerns, and she has begun to accept that further treatment would not improve the situation.

The relatives' needs for information

Establishing information needs is the same in principle for any individual (Chapter 5). However, there are particular points that have to be considered when meeting relatives' needs to be informed.

The role of the relative

We have already asked the question, 'Whose information?', and seen the problems that can arise if relatives are informed rather than the patient. What is certain is that most relatives (and indeed close friends) will wish to have some information about the condition and outlook of their loved one. It could be argued that this is not a concern of health professionals, since the patient can decide how much information he or she will share —and with whom.

Such rationalization is over-simplistic. Firstly, the patient may be in denial or unable to make sense of what he or she has been told. Secondly, it is very difficult to share bad news with those we love, so at best the assumption of the sharing of information will be over-optimistic. If the health professional can negotiate with the patient, there may be relief all round if relatives are informed by a member of the health-care team, at their own level of need.

Someone close to the patient may react to bad news with as much pain and grief as patients themselves. They may see their outlook as worse than that of the patient. Not for them the oblivion of death, but rather the pain of continued life after loss (Chapter 10).

Given such painful thoughts, it can be readily understood that some relatives respond to serious information with denial.

Denial

In Chapter 5 denial was put forward as a possible coping mechanism for patients who cannot come to terms with a poor prognosis. In relatives, a different approach must be taken, since *they* have to face the death of a loved one if they are going to grieve normally afterwards. Challenging any inconsistencies or looking for a window on denial to confront the relative with reality should be attempted, rather than a checking mechanism to discover if denial is complete. Challenging denial is discussed in more detail in Chapter 5.

Some relatives will have enormous difficulty in facing such a painful reality, especially if the dying patient is a much-loved child or partner. They may not readily accept the truth, and may indeed seek second opinions or alternative treatments for their beloved. The health professional who recognizes the relatives' problems and gives them time and space to talk through their feelings is more likely to help them face reality than the one who becomes impatient with false hopes of 'miracle cures'.

Hope

Just as patients need hope, so do relatives. Effective assessment will elicit the nature of these hopes and whether they are realistic. It is not easy for the professional, for so few promises can be made. Those that are made should be tempered with reality, so rather than saying, 'Of course we can promise that your mother will die pain-free,' we may have to say, 'We will do our best to keep her free from pain.' This avoids the justifiable anger, later, of people who feel cheated as they watch their mother's stormy death.

Relatives may still be angry, as they have to see hope fade, even if the professional has been realistic; but their anger may be more readily diffused by a nurse or a doctor who has earned trust, than by someone who has fed their unrealistic dreams.

Coping

When a situation is serious for a patient, as with aggressive therapy or impending death, it is important to monitor how the relatives are coping, and to ascertain whether they need help or advice. Sensitive assessment (Chapter 4) will elicit problems and give the relative a chance to discuss any associated feelings. This is an area which can be difficult, since the relative does not have to take advice. A common situation is that in which the mother of a dying child neglects the entire family to be with her child. She may not understand why her family expects some attention at such a time of crisis, and may not respond to the nurse or doctor who tries to persuade her to give family and herself some space. The professional can be firm, and point out that the current imbalance will have repercussions for the future; but the mother must be free to make her own informed choice within the family relationships.

A diagnosis of cancer, and the resultant uncertain future, may affect patient and relative in many different ways. Difficult relationships may be strengthened by the crisis, while apparently stable couples may find themselves divided. No assumptions can be made on how or why one person can cope while another is totally shattered by similar circumstances; but one fairly common reason for maintaining a 'brave face' may be the presence of children in the family.

Children

Normally, there is an overwhelming need on the part of parents to protect children from the pain of serious news about a parent, sibling, or other close relative. One rationalization is that of strong parent vs weak child, while another is that the child would be unable to deal with the concept of death. The result of these, and other, attitudes is that children are often excluded from the reality of illness and death, and may be prevented from attending the funeral of a figure formerly of great importance in their lives.

This protectiveness may have serious repercussions for a child who cannot understand why he or she has been left without a 'goodbye'. Because they have not seen the body or attended the funeral they may also have difficulties in believing that the beloved person will not return.

The reality is that even very young children can deal with serious illness and death if they are involved in a sensitive way. The following scenario illustrates this:

Joan and Alan knew that Joan was dying of cancer. She had cancer of the ovary with metastatic spread. From the outset their two children, Chris (7) and Duncan (5) had been told that Mummy was 'very tired' and 'needed to go to hospital from time to time to get well'. One night Alan awoke the boys and took them to stay at a friend's house, explaining that Mummy needed more rest. The children stayed at the friend's, and continued to go to school from there. Meanwhile, Joan died in hospital, and was cremated a few days later. After that, Alan collected the boys and took them home, when the following exchange took place.

Duncan:	Where is Mummy?
Alan:	Come here, both of you. I want you to be big, big boys.
Duncan:	*Where* is Mummy?
Chris:	[accusingly] She's dead, isn't she?
Duncan:	What's 'dead'?
Chris:	[crying] Daddy, I want Mummy.

Alan:	And she wants you, but she was very tired. She has gone to Heaven.
Duncan:	When will she come home?
Alan:	No, boys. Mummy can't come home. It's just us now.
Chris:	She left. She didn't say 'goodbye'. My friend said she was dead. I hit him.
Duncan:	[running up the stairs] Mummy! Mummy!

Such heartbreaking stories are not uncommon, nor are the consequent feelings of disbelief, in the absence of a body, or of abandonment and isolation that come from having been excluded from the family's reality. Obviously, while a patient is coping with illness, children need only be told that which squares with the reality that they can see. If the disease does not respond to treatment, then questions should be answered as they arise. Children are pragmatic, and their first question may be an aggrieved 'Why are you letting me down?' comment, such as 'Mummy, why are you always in bed? You promised to sew my badges on, *and* come to the barbecue?' Answers should be simple but honest, so that the child can begin to accept the concept of mortality. An answer to the above question such as 'Danny, I'd love to come to the barbecue, but I'm not very strong just now. I'll want you to tell me all about it later' may be accepted at face value, but may also generate more probing questions from the child.

Meeting children's needs in this way means that information is given at a level and rate to suit them. It is worth remembering that children, just like adults, will be attempting to make sense of the reality around them, and can be surprisingly accurate in their guesses.

If children are involved in this way they may well have grasped the fact that Mummy will *not* get better *before* the death occurs. This will not lessen their grief; but it will allow them to be part of the 'farewell' ritual along with other members of the family, and will almost certainly avoid the anger that arises from being excluded, which can have repercussions well into the future.

Summary

It can be seen in this chapter that relatives and those close to a patient cannot be excluded from the reality of cancer even when the outlook is good. They need to feel involved and considered as individuals, whereas so often they are seen as a faceless support network. Their vulnerability needs to be acknowledged, along with their need for support, even if giving such support means referral to other agencies.

10

Spiritual issues

In recent years, there has been an increase in concern about the spiritual care of patients who are suffering from fear-provoking diagnosis or prognosis. A major difficulty appears to be the interpretation of the phrase 'spiritual care'. At a basic level, it is interpreted as meaning that 'spiritual' equals 'religious'; but this over-simplifies a very important area. Stoter (1991) makes the point that 'So often spiritual care is seen as religious care for the few who request it and therefore becomes dismissed as a footnote.' By believing that spiritual care is tied in in some way with religion, it is very easy for health professionals to delegate such care and concern to members of the clergy.

The literal meaning of 'spiritual' is (i) 'essence' and (ii) 'chief quality'. This suggests that spirituality is much more to do with individuality and belief about oneself as a person than it is to do with religious beliefs, although they may be incorporated into a particular individual's view of her- or himself as a person. Many people would argue that they do not stop to analyse the 'essence' of themselves; but even those seemingly most unaware of their make-up and beliefs react quite strongly if they feel that they are being described in a way that does not fit with themselves as a person.

The effect of cancer on an individual's view of self
With few exceptions, for example smoking and lung cancer, there often is no clear reason why one individual should get cancer rather than another. With a lack of adequate explanation as to why an individual has been found to have cancer, there soon comes a search for meaning, meaning in terms of 'How can I explain what has happened to me?' There are two classic results of this search for meaning, guilt and anger, along with a variety of other responses.

Guilt

Many patients suffering from cancer, in trying to find a meaning in why cancer has attacked them rather than other people, look back into their past to find reasons why *they* have been punished. Few individuals lead a totally blameless life, so it is very easy for a patient to suffer from guilt. For example:

Fred: I can't think why I've got this cancer.
Nurse: Well, it's difficult to explain why some people get it and others don't.
Fred: Well, but it might be ...
Nurse: Yes.
Fred: Well, it was deliberate that we never had any children, and I'm a Catholic. I wonder if I'm being punished for that.

This attribution of cause and effect can extend to other members of the family. For example, in a study of childhood cancer (Faulkner *et al.* 1993) one father believed absolutely that his active service during the Suez crisis caused his child's cancer, and, for some years after the child was in remission, the father still walked down to the railway bridge and played with the idea of jumping over the bridge. Such guilt is difficult to dislodge; and indeed, sometimes the only people that can forgive people who feel that an act in their past caused their cancer are the individual him- or herself, with insight, or their religious adviser, if they have one, who can offer absolution through the rituals of prayers and formal blessings.

If people with cancer explain the disease in terms of some past misdeed, they are then having to handle a change in their view of themselves as individuals acceptable to others. The belief that a past experience has been so bad as to warrant a punishment as shattering as cancer may indeed make the individual believe that he or she is no longer acceptable to friends and family. This issue, if it is not raised and discussed, can become very large in terms of its importance to the patient. Those who observe the patient, and are not aware of the sense that he or she is making of what is going on, may be concerned by what appears to be silent distress. In this situation, careful assessment is required to discover what sense the individual *is* making of his or her cancer and current situation, and to identify the resultant problems.

Anger

It is not unusual for spiritual distress to present as anger. It was seen in Chapter 7 that anger is not an uncommon reaction to a diagnosis of cancer. An important element of being oneself is the feeling that one has control over one's life and what goes on in it, to a large extent. Patients with cancer may often feel that their control of their life has been taken from them by the disease. They don't know how it came, why it's there, or, often, what effect it will have on their abilities and their image during the remainder of their life. In those circumstances, anger may be seen as a natural response, but nevertheless one that needs to be explored with the patient through careful assessment. In working with the anger, it is often possible to move the patient on to a transition from the anger to the feelings surrounding that anger.

Jane: [angrily] Everything was working out so well, and now *this*.

Doctor: What do you mean by 'this'?

Jane: Well, my life isn't my own. I've got no control any more of what I do or where I go; up and down to the hospital; one test after another; treatment that makes me feel so lousy: I've just had enough.

Doctor: Sounds as if you feel it's all very unfair.

Jane: Yes; yes it is. I just can't take it any more.

[later]

Jane: I'm sorry, doctor, I shouldn't take it out on you; but, you know, things all looked so well, and now I'll never see little Mary grow up; and I'm sad because I can't any longer be to her what I've loved being.

In the above sequence, because Jane was allowed to defuse her anger she made the transition to her true emotions of sadness that she could no longer be the grandmother she had been. The main element here is the disclosure of the frustration experienced through loss of control and the feeling that other people are making the decisions, rather than the patient herself.

Sometimes the anger surrounding spiritual distress is self-directed, though this may not be immediately apparent. When anger is self-directed it is very often linked with feelings of guilt, and in those cases the health carer needs to be able to help the patient deal with both emotions. When spirituality includes religious belief, anger is very often directed at the individual's God, being generated by a sense of betrayal. People with religious upbringing and beliefs find it very hard to equate a God of love with someone who could send a life-threatening illness, seemingly without any clearly identifiable cause, and often to individuals who are young or are seen to be special in some way.

The above response needs to be dealt with in the same way as any other anger; but the individual concerned may feel that it would help to talk through the religious problems with a member of the clergy. In this respect, it is the health professionals' responsibility to identify the problems through careful assessment, but to refer on if they themselves do not feel able to deal with religious matters.

Reactions from others
In accepting the notion that spirituality is the essence and the chief quality of an individual, it becomes important to consider not only how individuals view themselves and what their beliefs about themselves are, but also the way that others perceive them, whether family, friends, or colleagues, in both social and work settings.

Many people believe that cancer equals death, and, in Western culture at least, death is still largely a taboo subject. The reactions of patients to their diagnosis and prognosis will not only be linked to their own belief system, but will also be coloured by the reactions of those whom they love. If, for example, friends and relatives start to avoid patients, they may feel that they are no longer acceptable as individuals, and may be experiencing spiritual distress. It is hard for a patient, who already has much to bear, to understand that the reactions of others are often due to myths, ignorance, and embarrassment that are all brought into play once they know that their loved one has cancer.

Patients are generally very loyal to partners and family members; but if distress is identified and found to belong in the arena of the patient's social life, then steps can be taken, firstly, to help the patient realize that the avoidance behaviour is not necessarily personal to the patient, but may be much more associated with feelings engendered by the cancer. And secondly, it may be necessary to talk to a relative and find out what the problem is:

Nurse:	Mr Smith, I wonder if I could have a word with you about your wife?
Mr Smith:	All right, sister.
Nurse:	I wonder how you think she is just now?
Mr Smith:	Oh, she's pretty upset most of the time. I think she wonders what's going to happen to her.
Nurse:	And how do you feel?
Mr Smith:	Well, I guess I'm the last person who can help her. I simply don't know what to say to her.
Nurse:	Can you tell me what you mean by that?

Mr Smith:	Well, I come in at visiting times. It's quite obvious she's not really interested in the sort of things I talk about, like my mates at work and how I'm managing at home.
Nurse:	And ...
Mr Smith:	Well, I know she wants to talk about being ill, and she tried the other day to talk about the future; but I can't handle it, I'm sorry.
Nurse:	Is there any way we can help you to handle it?
Mr Smith:	Well, I suppose if I knew more about it—but it isn't just that. I can't bear the thought of anything happening to her.

In the above sequence it can be seen that although Mrs Smith was distressed that her husband seemed to be avoiding having a reasonable conversation with her, Mr Smith himself needed considerable help before he could be in any way able to meet his wife's needs.

It is often easy to forget that cancer may bring a new and frightening dimension to the lives of both the patient and those who are close to the patient. They may have no previous experience of talking about a foreshortened future, or about an unknown type of death, and may literally not know what to talk about (Buckman 1988). By exploring these issues with the relatives it may be possible to help them to gain some level of acceptance of the current situation, so that they can at least have a dialogue with their loved one. The help they may need may include not only knowledge of their loved one's particular disease, treatment, and outlook, but also help in understanding the whole notion of cancer; and possibly they may need some help in basing their beliefs on fact rather than misconceptions.

One popular misconception is that cancer is catching. If someone believes this, then they are likely to treat patients as if they were not acceptable. They may show this in avoidance behaviour and in definite obvious distancing techniques. This type of behaviour can lead patients to question their own beliefs about themselves, for if those that they love suddenly don't want to talk to them or appear not to want to be with them, this can cause considerable concern to the patient about his or her self-image. If, for example, a patient is feeling guilty and believing himself or herself to have been given cancer as punishment for past misdeeds, the behaviour of his or her relatives will fit in with that concept of non-acceptability, and this can lead to considerable spiritual distress.

These feelings can lead to a frightening sense of isolation—a major cause of spiritual distress—as the patient reacts by suppressing true feelings of fear, confusion, pain, and guilt. This can extend to professional carers unless they have the skills to encourage the patient to disclose in a non-judgemental way.

Taking over

Problems may also arise for the very different reason of the relatives' becoming over-protective. We have seen that a common manifestation of protecting the patient is to collude in such a way that the patient is kept in ignorance of the true diagnosis and prognosis. The need to protect a loved one who has cancer can also lead to attempts to do too much for them, thus heightening the feeling of loss of control on the part of the patient. Miss Jellie had lived with her female friend, Miss McArthur, for thirty years. They bred dogs in a desultory way, and had a very nice life together, in which Miss McArthur took the more decisive role. When she subsequently contracted cancer and became very ill, Miss Jellie took over the mothering role for her friend, and made decisions on what was best in terms of fighting the cancer. This 'role reversal' caused enormous problems in their relationship, because Miss McArthur did not wish to adopt the same approach to her disease as her friend, but because she was feeling so ill she was unable to articulate her true feelings to her friend.

Miss Jellie's action was born out of kindness and concern, but caused enormous spiritual distress to her friend, who felt that the person that she had always thought she was suddenly did not exist any more.

Facing death

When the patient with advanced cancer faces the reality of impending death, these questions of 'me as a person' often become more pressing. Most people who are well do not face their own mortality. It is only when a crisis arises that threatens one's future that questions about the after-life and what happens to the 'me that I believe I am' arise. These reactions in patients may cause problems for health professionals as they come face to face with their own mortality.

It can be seen from the above that this may be a very frightening time for an individual, no matter what label we put on the concerns expressed. Whether the issues are indeed spiritual or largely existential, they do need to be addressed. This can cause problems for health professionals, depending on their own belief systems, and it can be as worrying for the patient to be faced with a health professional with strong religious beliefs as to be faced with one with no beliefs at all. Note the following exchanges:

A.

Jack: Nurse, do you think there's anything after this?

Nurse: After this?

Jack: Yeah, you know, Heaven, St Peter at the gate, and all that sort of thing. Do you think there is something else, or is there just going to be a day when there's no more Jack anywhere?

Nurse: Jack, I thought you were a good Christian. You've been to the church service every Sunday since you've been here.

Jack: I know all that, but I've got a lot of questions, and my time is short.

Nurse: You shouldn't need to ask questions Jack, you just need to believe, and then everything will be all right.

B.

Nurse: Jack, Jack.

Jack: Sorry nurse, I was miles away. I was just wondering what there is after this.

Nurse: What do you mean by that?

Jack: Well, do you reckon there is a Heaven, and there is St Peter waiting at the gate, and all my sins will be forgiven?

Nurse: Jack, I can see how worried you are by these concerns; but I'm not the best person to help you. I hope there is, but I honestly don't know. I wonder if there's anybody else who could help you.

Jack: I don't think there is. I talked to the minister last Sunday; and, well, nobody can make any promises, can they?

Nurse: No; I'm sorry I can't help you.

Jack: Well, it does help to talk about it, and not to be told to have a prayer, because I think I'm at the end of prayer.

In the above exchange, Jack, whose religious faith had been badly shaken by his cancer, was having to accept that no one can answer questions about what happens next. In the first exchange he was made to feel guilty for his lack of faith in his God: but in the second he was allowed to explore his feelings, with no judgements being made about his failing beliefs. Occasionally this is the most that the health professional can do for people who are questioning the beliefs that they have held about themselves and their world for a lifetime.

Assessment

It was seen in Chapter 3 that assessing a patient's concerns is of major importance in planning care and meeting needs. This assessment includes identifying concerns which can be seen to have a spiritual base. In this area particularly, the importance of being non-judgemental cannot be overstated. For example, when the nurse suggested to Jack that he should pray and renew his faith, she was in fact reiterating his growing belief that the 'essence' of him had somehow changed. If people are to die with dignity, they need to die with their beliefs about themselves and their world as intact as possible, and with the belief that they are not responsible either for their cancer or its consequences, unless that is in fact the case.

Assessing spiritual distress requires that patients are given a chance to express concerns about themselves, their responsibilities, and, sometimes, the deeper meaning of life. This part of assessment can be very painful for patients as they explore their feelings, so health professionals need to give patients the space to identify those areas of major concern without influencing them or making them feel that somehow a different attitude to life on their part could have avoided the current situation.

In this situation, patients who have a cancer with a known cause, as with for example lung cancer and smoking, seem to have fewer problems in identifying spiritual issues. For them, there is a known and accepted cause, so they do not have to look for other more complex reasons for their situation that might throw doubt on themselves as the people whom they have always believed themselves to be. This does not mean that there will not be spiritual issues arising; but there is likely to be less guilt, and more acceptance of cause and effect. There may still be a questioning of beliefs, particularly their religious beliefs about God and love, in the face of seemingly senseless harm.

Relieving spiritual distress

When distress is identified that is linked to an individual's belief system, it is not always possible to alleviate that distress. As with other difficult issues, it is important to acknowledge the concerns of the patient, and, where possible, to make those concerns legitimate, for example:

Mavis: You know, doctor, I've never had any very strong religious beliefs, but I've always felt that I knew where

	I was in my world and I knew where I was going; and suddenly I don't any more. It's as if what I believed about myself doesn't hold true.
Doctor:	That must be very difficult for you.
Mavis:	Yes, the thoughts just go round and round in my mind, and I wonder if there is anything different that I could have done that would have saved me from this.
Doctor:	Is there any way that we can help you here?
Mavis:	I don't know; I just feel so totally out of control.

Mavis had two problems—one was accepting her current situation with equanimity, and the second was needing to regain some control over her life that she felt had been eroded by the cancer. Although carers cannot always offer answers, the recognition and acceptance of spiritual distress can help to relieve feelings of isolation.

Acceptance

Acceptance is seen as a final stage of working through the reality that life is foreshortened. Kubler-Ross (1969) suggests stages that patients work through when they are coming to grips with the reality of death. This paradigm is useful as a concept, but is often interpreted as something that must happen to everyone. As a result, all patients are expected to be shocked and horrified by their diagnosis, and to work through a number of stages, including anger and bargaining, to a final stage of acceptance.

In reality, there are more individual reactions. For example, many individuals are born angry and die angry, and some may never reach the level of acceptance required if the person is to die in mental peace. What the health professional can do is to give the patient the opportunity to explore fears and worries and to work through for themselves as much as is possible in order to accept the reality of what is happening. This process may be linked with working through guilt, anger, and the other many emotions which may arise. Strategies for helping patients achieve this are given in other chapters of the book.

Since some of the concerns that the dying patient has may be linked to the attitudes of others, particularly much-loved others, the patient may be helped if an open dialogue can be initiated between the patient and his or her family. This may require separate assessment of relatives, and occasionally reveal the need to bring the parties together in order to get a dialogue started. Such a dialogue may be quite painful for all concerned, but may well clear the path to reinforcement by others of the proposition that the patient remains his or her own person with his or her own personality and 'essence'. What the health professional is offering here is support and concern.

Control

Many patients are much more able to face impending death if they feel that as far as possible they are in control of the situation. They will look to several areas where they feel that control has been taken from them: for example, the health professional who is dictating treatment and care, and/or family members who are over-protective and over-zealous in attempting to alleviate the patient's distress.

It may not always be possible for individuals to regain total control of their lives. Physical disability may get in the way, as may social problems; but what can be most helpful is that others should encourage patients to identify the areas in which they feel that they have been taken over. Too often both the health professional and the family members feel that they know what is best for the patient, without properly assessing the situation. In this, one of the most important areas to many patients is that they maintain some sense of personal space. The dying patient is often exhausted by over-visiting and too much love. Because of the emotive aspects of being terminally ill, people are often far too polite to each other, but at the same time not really comfortable with the situation that they are in. They may need to express negative emotions and responses.

A common practice in the Western world is based on the belief that individuals should not die alone. As a result, long vigils are kept by the patient's bed, usually by a close friend or partner. The frequency with which the patient dies in the short space of time in which the loved one has left to have a meal, a bath, or whatever, suggests that right to the end dying patients may wish for some control over what they do. Although there is no scientific proof, it would appear that dying patients may often choose to die when other people have left them alone in peace for a short time.

Summary

It has been seen in this chapter that the whole area of spirituality is one that is not fully understood. It appears to be related to individuals' beliefs about themselves, the 'essence' of themselves, and the qualities of the person that they are, whether or not these include religious beliefs. It has been seen that the invasion of cancer without the control of the patient can cause questions about spirituality in terms of self-value and punishment. Guilt and anger are common elements of spiritual distress, plus the feeling of control being taken by others.

It has been suggested that spiritual distress should be as carefully assessed as any other aspect of a patient's concerns; that such distress should be acknowledged, and made legitimate if this is appropriate; and that efforts should be made to meet patients' needs to reinstate their beliefs in themselves as persons. This includes the restoration of control and a working, as far as possible, towards accepting that the situation has not been self-made.

References

Buckman, R. (1988). *I don't know what to say*. Macmillan, London.

Kubler-Ross, E. (1969). *On death and dying*. Souvenir Press, London.

Faulkner, A., Peace, G., and O'Keeffe, C. (1993). Future imperfect. *Nursing Times*, **89** (51), 40–3.

Stoter, D. (1991). Spiritual care. In *Palliative care for people with cancer* (ed. J. Penson and R. Fisher), pp. 187–98. Edward Arnold, London.

11

Assessing the bereaved

Introduction

Most people who lose a close friend or relative through cancer find the strength to cope with it from within and from others close to them, and are able to grieve normally. However, a substantial minority fail to cope, and are at risk of psychiatric and physical illness.

Consequences of unresolved grief

The failure to grieve normally is associated with an increased risk of psychiatric and physical morbidity. The psychiatric morbidity includes generalized anxiety disorder, depressive illness, alcoholism, hypochondriasis, and agoraphobia (Parkes 1965). The development of depression and alcoholism, separately or in combination, is associated with an increased risk of suicide. The risk of suicide continues for up to eight years after bereavement, particularly at the time of important anniversaries like birthdays or weddings.

Failure to grieve normally also has longer-term consequences. It makes the individual more vulnerable to subsequent loss and at greater risk of developing mental illness when experiencing other stressful life events which threaten some form of loss, for example of job or role.

The loss of a parent in early life has also been found to have long-term effects in respect of an individual's vulnerability to life events (Brown and Harris 1978). Moreover, it may have a negative effect on an individual's ability to form and maintain relationships. A person who experienced sudden abandonment in childhood through the loss of a parent and the lack of an adequate replacement person may become fearful, when he or she begins a relationship, that such abandonment will occur again. She or he can either, therefore, avoid relationships getting to any emotional depth, or become 'clingy' and dependent for fear that he or she will lose the other person. This clinging and dependent behaviour may drive the other person away, and so provoke a severe depressive illness.

It has been found that there is an increased risk of death from heart disease in spouses within the first six months after bereavement (Parkes *et al.* 1969). Relatives of people who died suddenly, unexpectedly, and away from home are also at risk of dying from heart disease, although the aetiology of this is unclear. Older people are more prone to developing arthritic diseases.

Given the psychiatric and physical morbidity, it is important to be able to distinguish normal from abnormal grief and to know when to intervene to help an individual to resolve the bereavement.

Normal grief

If someone is to grieve normally, he or she has to have realized that death has occurred and acknowledge this intellectually and emotionally. When the individual was present at the time of death, the period of numbness or shock should last only a few hours or a few days. Then the onset of grief should be obvious. It should include intrusive waves of very strong feelings such as a sense of loss, sadness, or despair. Other feelings commonly experienced and expressed include anger, guilt, and feelings of loneliness and emptiness. Often these feelings come together, which leads the bereaved person to talk in terms of feeling 'confused'. Between these strong waves of feelings, the person feels either calm or apathetic.

Over the next few days after death, particularly after the funeral, these waves of grief escalate in their frequency, duration, and intensity until they reach a natural plateau. Here the individual is grieving maximally, but is not feeling in danger of 'going mad' or being 'overwhelmed' by it.

Other mental accompaniments of grieving include a strong sense of the presence of the dead person. This is often comforting, but can provoke a realization that the person is no longer there and waves of grief. The bereaved may experience an illusion where they perceive that somebody looks like the dead person, but then realize that this is an illusion. Some people experience actual hallucinations, in which they insist that they have seen or heard the dead person. Such hallucinations are natural in the early weeks after death.

Some individuals become concerned when they find themselves pacing restlessly within the house going from room to room or find they are going to places where they might have expected to find the dead person alive. For example, a mother who has lost a child might find herself going past the school gate. These behaviours represent searching that is designed to try and make contact with the dead person.

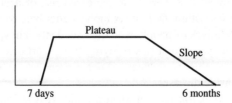

Fig. 11.1 Normal grief.

Feelings of anxiety, depression, and ideas of suicide can occur, but are usually sporadic and do not persist. Nor do they result in the person formulating any clear suicidal plans. Similarly, feelings of irritability, poor concentration, and poor memory are common but fleeting in the early stages.

Recently bereaved people also experience a number of physical symptoms, including for example palpitations, chest pain, dizziness, feeling drained, and various aches and pains. Given the risk of heart disease it is important to take any symptoms suggestive of that seriously and investigate the patient.

In most individuals the period of maximum grief will last some eight to twelve weeks. Then the individual will notice that the waves of grief have become less frequent, of less duration, and less intense, though still occurring. Thus normal grief can be represented in diagrammatic form (Fig. 11.1). Once this slope is developed it can take a considerable time for the slope to return to normal, though it usually does so within the year.

Markers of normal grief
The key feature is that normally grieving individuals are able to accept emotionally that their loved one is dead. They are able to express their grief, and develop a slope within a reasonable time interval. They are able to get rid of the belongings, apart from holding on to important mementoes. They are able to connect with good memories of the deceased, and are able to visit the cemetery or crematorium and express their distress, but only attend at sensible intervals. They are able to look at photographs, and were able to attend the funeral or cremation and face the moment when the coffin went below the surface of the ground or behind the curtains. The amount of time they spend thinking about the dead person has clearly lessened, as have the phenomena of searching or experiencing illusions and hallucinations. This is illustrated by the experience of Mrs Short.

Mrs Short lost her husband from bowel cancer. He was admitted to hospital six weeks before his death, but surgery proved ineffective. He had been ill for some months before admission, and Mrs Short was aware that he was likely to die from his disease. They had had a very good relationship together, and they had been able to reappraise their life together and say important things to each other before he died. Although his death still came as a shock, she realized and accepted that he was dead and the doctor's explanation of the cause. Within a few hours she felt extremely upset and began to grieve. The waves of grief were intense, but she was able to function from day to day until the funeral. She was able to attend the funeral, although she found it very upsetting and cried a great deal, both during the service and particularly at the graveside when the coffin was lowered below the surface of the ground. She found the moment when she had to throw soil on the coffin especially distressing. However, at that point she was able to say good-bye to him and reiterate how much she loved him.

Over the next few weeks she continued to grieve, and the waves of grief came on a regular basis. After three to four months, however, they began to lessen in frequency, amplitude, and duration.

She was able to visit the cemetery fortnightly. Although she felt sad when she was by the graveside, she could connect with good times they had had together and feel comforted.

She was able to get rid of his clothes and other belongings, but kept a watch and other important mementoes to remind her of him and the good times they had had. She kept photographs of him so that they were visible, and was able to look at them and feel comforted, though sometimes they triggered further waves of grief. Over time, as the waves of grief lessened, she felt less preoccupied with thoughts of him, and was able to return to work. Throughout her bereavement she was able to share her feelings and experiences with friends and colleagues who were supportive to her, both practically and emotionally.

She became aware of the 'big hole' which his death had left in her life, and began to realize the need to take up new activities to fill the void. These included joining a drama class and taking up golf. She still misses him considerably, and can be distressed occasionally, but she feels that life must go on and that he would support her in her endeavour to forge a new life.

Abnormal grief
It is important to recognize abnormal patterns of grief because of their association in the later psychiatric disorders.

Absent grief

In absent grief there is no evidence of grief developing, despite the reality of death. The individual is either denying the death on 'automatic', or actively blocking the reality because it is too painful. There is often evidence of this in the account of early reactions to bereavement.

Mrs Halton was a 35-year-old teacher whose husband worked as a policeman. They had a good relationship, and he was very supportive of her. He was interested in sports and fond of athletics. Throughout their life together he had been healthy. One day he came home and complained that he was experiencing pain in his stomach. They both thought that the most likely explanation was that this was an ulcer. He went to see his General Practitioner immediately, who examined him and said he thought it was an ulcer, but advised that he see a specialist. When he saw the specialist within the next week, the specialist warned him that although it was probably an ulcer it could be more serious, and that he would like him in immediately for further investigation. The result of the investigations was that he was found to have advanced cancer of the stomach, with widespread metastases. He and his wife were told together. He was admitted to hospital, but died within two weeks of admission.

Mrs Halton found it impossible to accept that a man who had been so well and had so few symptoms could have died. She could not face seeing him at the point of death or after death, and insisted on the possibility that he was alive somewhere. She refused to attend the Chapel of Rest, and although she was able to attend the funeral she described it as 'happening to somebody else'. When she saw the coffin she could not accept that her husband was in it. She refused to go to the graveside for the actual burial. Six months after his death she still refused to believe he had gone.

She kept his belongings in exactly the same places, because she believed he would come back at some point. She did not take down the photographs. She did not see any point in visiting the cemetery, because her husband was not buried there. She continued to behave as though he were alive, and set the table each evening. When relatives pointed out how inappropriate this was, she insisted she had to do it in case he came back. Six months after his death she was still talking about him in the present tense ('he is'). This form of abnormal grief is illustrated in Fig. 11.2.

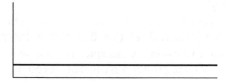

Fig. 11.2 Absent grief.

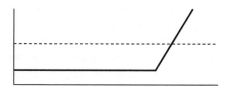

Fig. 11.3 Delayed grief.

Delayed grief

Delayed grief shows a similar pattern to absent grief, except that the individual makes a conscious and successful effort to avoid grieving. They may argue that they have to carry on with life because of a need to continue their job or because of the needs of family members. So they consider they do not have time to grieve. However, these reasons may be alibis that allow them to avoid facing their grief, which they sense will be just too painful. When grief is delayed like this it is very difficult for other members of the family, for example children, to feel free to grieve themselves. Such delay can be maintained for some time, but grief is usually triggered by some strong reminder of the dead person.

Mrs Dobson's husband died of lung cancer. They had been happily married for fifteen years. Mrs Dobson felt she had to keep going for the sake of her two children (Mandy, 7, and Susan, 5). When she attended the funeral she felt that it would be upsetting if she broke down, and close friends and relatives commented on her tranquil demeanour. In response to a friend's enquiry she snapped 'Grief, I've no time for grief. The girls need a caring mother, not a weeping widow.' Subsequently Mrs Dobson found she could not get in touch with her grief, and sought help. She was advised to take time out by asking her mother to look after the children and seeing a therapist, who was able to put her in touch with her true feelings. A normal pattern of grieving then emerged.

Delayed grief is illustrated in Fig. 11.3.

Oscillating grief

Here the individual allows the grief to emerge reasonably soon after the bereavement, but soon realizes that the grief is too painful to risk allowing it full expression. Consequently, the individual actively suppresses the grief and pushes it back. This succeeds only for a short time, and the grief emerges again, only to be suppressed again. This suppression takes a huge amount of mental energy. Before long, usually in a few months, the individual runs out of reserves. When that happens the grief not only emerges but tends to explode, and to go rapidly beyond the normal plateau. This usually provokes considerable anxiety and major depression, and constitutes an emergency.

Mrs Foulds had a three-year-old daughter who was diagnosed as having a retinoblastoma, a tumour of the eye. She was particularly bitter at the time of diagnosis because she had taken the child on several occasions to the General Practitioner, who had said she could see nothing wrong with the child's vision. Later it became clear that the tumour could have been diagnosed earlier. This was confirmed by the hospital to whom the child was referred. Despite various treatments, the tumour spread aggressively. Not only did it lead her to becoming blind in that eye, but it also invaded her mouth. Consequently Mrs Foulds had to witness her daughter becoming mutilated and struggling to eat and swallow. After eighteen months of ineffective treatment, with many visits to hospital, her daughter died.

The daughter was her first child, after many years of trying to have a baby. She had developed an extremely close bond with her, and found it intolerably painful to consider that she had died in such an awful way. Every time she began to think about her after her death, the images of her suffering physically and emotionally were uppermost.

Because these images were so painful, she tried actively to suppress them and the associated feelings of grief. Each time her grief feelings emerged she worked actively to 'swallow them back' or 'stop thinking about them'. She felt that people around her did not understand how awful it had been for her to lose her child in this way, particularly as her husband opted out of responsibility. Instead of helping her through this period he spent more time away from the house, usually by drinking in the local public house.

After four months, she ran out of reserves and could no longer suppress her feelings. Her grief escalated beyond the plateau, and she became suicidally depressed. This led to her being admitted as a psychiatric emergency. Her wish for suicide was provoked by a wish to escape the torment of her suffering, particularly the images of her daughter's suffering and death, and a wish to join her dead daughter.

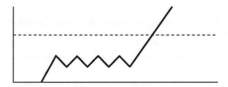

Fig. 11.4 Oscillating grief.

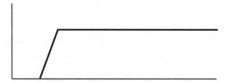

Fig. 11.5 Chronic grief.

Throughout this period she was unable to visit the cemetery where her daughter was buried, because she realized it would be too painful. She was unable to get rid of the child's belongings, including her toys, because she felt it would be like 'throwing my daughter away'. She could not look at photographs, because they induced intolerable pain, though she was not able to move them either. Oscillating grief is illustrated in Fig. 11.4.

Chronic grief
Here the grief usually develops normally, and moves on to the optimal plateau. However, there is no evidence of any slope developing, even after months or years. The individual continues to experience all the signs and symptoms of grieving. Commonly, when assessed, they can talk about their grief at length, but they do not allow themselves to express fully the underlying feelings. Such chronic grief is usually accompanied by a history of avoidance. Thus they will report that they were reluctant to see the person at the point of death or in the Chapel of Rest, or to attend the funeral. They also tend to avoid visiting the cemetery, looking at photographs, and getting rid of belongings. The overall impression is that they are trying to 'hang on' to the dead person and avoid letting go, usually because of a deep underlying fear of emptiness and desolation. Chronic grief is illustrated in Fig. 11.5.

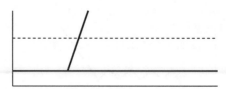

Fig. 11.6 Exploding grief.

Exploding grief

Here the grief develops within normal time-limits, but then accelerates beyond the normal plateau. The individual then feels overwhelmed with feelings, and often expresses a fear of 'going crazy'.

Mr Winter had a daughter who was eighteen years old. She had been diagnosed two years previously as having a sarcoma of her left leg. She underwent an amputation, and seemed to be responding well to surgery followed by chemotherapy. Mr Winter had invested a lot of hope and ambition in her because she was intelligent and likely to go to university. He felt strongly that he had had no such opportunities during his own childhood. When her sarcoma returned he was devastated, particularly as the doctors indicated that it could preclude her going to university. However, they advised a further course of chemotherapy. This had serious side-effects, and led to his daughter losing her hair and much weight. He was extremely upset at the change in her appearance, and worried about what he perceived to be her loss of dignity. Even so, she responded to treatment, and was able to begin her university course.

Six months after going to university, her sarcoma returned yet again, and failed to respond to treatment. Mr Winter felt very angry that somebody with such a future should have been deprived of it. Within a few days of her death, he was inconsolable, and had started drinking heavily. It was the only way he could tranquillize the terrible feelings that were emerging. He felt guilty that he had been unable to guarantee that his daughter achieved a healthy adulthood. His grief escalated beyond the normal plateau, and he became suicidal. This pattern of grief is illustrated in Fig. 11.6.

Markers of abnormal grief

Here, the individual is unable to accept, at an emotional level, that the person has died. They will usually avoid being present at the time of death, and will try to avoid seeing the dead person in the Chapel of Rest. If they do so, they will be unable to accept that the person is real. They will try to avoid attending the funeral or cremation.

They will find it difficult to get rid of the belongings, and will tend to hide them all away. They may even go to the extent of maintaining a room as a shrine, in the hope that the dead person will return. They may either put many photographs up around the house, or hide them all away because they are too painful. They may avoid going to the cemetery or crematorium, or they may spend an excessive amount of time going, and explain that they are maintaining contact with the dead person and having conversations with him or her. They may even be tempted to dig up the dead person.

There will be no evidence of a slope being established. Instead they will continue to complain either of an absence of grief, an excess of grief, or continuous grief, without any let up in the frequency, amplitude, or duration of the waves of feeling. They will continue to be preoccupied, both in their waking time and their sleep, with thoughts of the dead person. This will not have lessened over time. They will continue to experience a strong sense of the presence of the dead person, illusions, and hallucinations. They will usually complain that they cannot connect with good memories of the dead person. Instead they are plagued with memories of unpleasant events surrounding the person's death or its aftermath.

Risk factors
It has been found that certain factors carry a high risk of an individual developing an abnormal grief reaction.

Nature of relationships
Individuals who have a very strong but mutual dependence on each other are particularly at risk. For they have not needed to turn to other friends for support or comfort at times of crisis, and have been self-sufficient as a couple.

Similarly, individuals who are over-dependent on the other person are left abandoned when that individual dies. They may never have had to make important day-to-day decisions in life or to take responsibility. They are therefore ill-prepared for the sudden and unwanted autonomy.

Those who had stormy relationships and felt very ambivalent, in that they both loved and hated the dead person, can find that guilt feelings block the emergence of their grief. For at some time they would have wished their partner dead.

Some individuals develop a skew relationship. For example, a woman may have a reasonable relationship with her husband, but may sense there is something lacking. A child is then born who has a sparkling personality and who is very loving. She then turns increasingly to this child for emotional satisfaction. When this child becomes ill and later dies she feels extremely bitter and angry, because the most important person in her life has been taken from her. By this time she will have become distanced and decoupled from her partner, and so will not get the necessary support. Such skew relationships can lead to profound psychiatric problems after bereavement.

Mrs Taylor had a marriage that she thought was reasonably happy until she gave birth to a son. He proved a lively personality who liked to cuddle her and make her feel good. This made her aware that her marriage was lacking in certain respects. Unfortunately, when this boy reached his teenage years he developed leukaemia. He had a stormy illness, with several relapses and adverse side-effects from chemotherapy. She had to spend an increasing amount of time with him, with the result that she neglected her husband and the rest of her family. Her last memories of him were of his being extremely ill, suffering from septicaemia and haemorrhaging in the intensive care unit.

During his illness she had felt unsupported by the family, her friends, and the hospital staff, since they expected her to do a great deal for her son, including some basic nursing.

After her son's death she became angry that the most important person in her life had been taken from her. She developed a severe depressive illness, and made a serious attempt to kill herself in order to escape the torment and join her dead son.

Circumstances of death

Death which is sudden and unexpected and takes a violent form is especially hard to come to terms with, especially if the grieving person is not able to witness the body. Thus a woman who had emigrated to Canada learned that her son had a brain tumour and had been admitted to a local cancer hospital in England. Before she could get the necessary air fare together and make travel arrangements, she had a telephone call to say he had died. Moreover, she was told that he experienced a series of epileptic fits before he died, because of the effect of the brain tumour. She found that she was increasingly preoccupied with images of how much he must have suffered in the few days before his death, particularly when he was 'fitting'. She also felt guilty that she was not able to be there at the time of death.

It is important to know whether a death could have been prevented either by the person who has been bereaved or by other people like health professionals. For it can be hard to accept a death when the grieving person believes it need not have happened, as in the following example.

Mrs Ash was concerned that her daughter had developed a breast lump, and pressed her to seek help. Her daughter saw a surgeon, who advised her that the lump was benign and she needed no further help. The daughter believed this, and even though the symptoms changed in nature she still considered that she had a benign lump. The mother pressed her to seek further help, but she was reluctant to do so because she had a holiday coming up. Some weeks later she consulted a surgeon, who then told her that she had cancer and that she had to have a mastectomy. By this time the lymph nodes were involved, and her prognosis was poor.

The mother found it difficult to accept her death for two reasons. First she was worried that when her daughter presented initially the cancer might have been present. Second, she was concerned that her daughter delayed in seeking help when the symptoms changed. Guilt about her own inaction and anger at her daughter made it difficult for her to deal with her grief. She is still struggling with it some five years later.

A major issue is whether people have sufficient reserves to cope with the trauma of bereavement. This will be less likely if they have had to nurse the dead person for a long time and the illness has been stormy. They are likely to be left with unpleasant images because they spent so much time in face-to-face contact with the dead person, and may have watched a person they loved waste away in front of them.

Time of death
It is much harder to accept a death if the person who is surviving is left with considerable unfinished emotional and practical business. This is especially true when the bereaved person realizes that important ambitions, like having children or grandchildren, have been thwarted. Death occurring when a positive outcome was expected (for example a man losing his fiancée through leukaemia six months before their marriage) can be especially difficult to accept and work through. Similarly, the death of a young person in adolescence can cause great difficulties. For this is often a time of great rebellion, and the parents are struggling to work through this. They can be left feeling bewildered and guilty.

Lack of perceived support

A major factor that helps people grieve is a feeling that other people understand and support them in their predicament. So if people complain that they are not getting such support, this complaint should be heeded and attempts should be made to remedy the situation.

Other life crises

When people are having to cope with other major problems at a time of bereavement, for example, problems with finance, housing, or un-employment, they may not have the additional energy to deal with the bereavement.

Competing responsibilities

Some people believe they have to keep going for the sake of their business, job, or family, and do not allow themselves time out to grieve. However, it is important to be aware that this can be used as an alibi to allow the individual deliberately to avoid the real pain of bereavement.

Assessment of the recently bereaved

A key question is who should be assessed. Since most people grieve normally after the death of a relative from cancer, there is no need to assess everybody. However, any person who has disclosed any of those risk factors that have been discussed should be monitored within one to two months after bereavement. This can be done by any health professional with the necessary assessment skills.

There is the possibility that some of those who have no risk factors may have great difficulties resolving their bereavement. So it is useful to offer the bereaved an invitation along the following lines: 'I hope everything will be all right for you despite what has happened. It is clearly going to be painful for you. If things begin to be a real struggle please get in touch with me so that I can assess how you are and determine if we need to offer you any help.'

Most relatives can be relied upon to respond constructively to such an invitation, rather than abuse it by making undue demands on the health professional.

This approach enables assessments to be concentrated on those who are most likely to need help. It also allows families to utilize their own resources to resolve their grief, rather than turning to health professionals.

Mode of assessment

You should begin by negotiation.

Dr Green:	I would like to talk to you about the death of your daughter, Emily. I realize that this could be very upsetting for you, so I would like to check that you are prepared to talk about it before we go any further.
Mrs Stevens:	I know it could be painful, but I realize it might help me.

Once the bereaved person has agreed to discuss the bereavement, it is important to try and help her connect with her memories and experiences of the bereavement by encouraging her to be precise about what happened.

Dr Green:	Do you mind telling me exactly when Emily died? What exactly happened?
Mrs Stevens:	She died last August the 15th. She had been very ill for a few days, and drifted into coma.

Beginning such an account can be very painful. The bereaved person may look increasingly distressed or try to suppress any feelings. It is important then to renegotiate her preparedness to continue.

If the person is prepared to allow this, you should use every opportunity to explore feelings, since the active expression of grief is critical.

Dr Green:	How did you feel when Emily drifted into coma?
Mrs Stevens:	I realized it was getting to the end.
Dr Green:	How did that leave you feeling?
Mrs Stevens:	Feeling devastated. She was our only child; she had no right to die at such a young age.
Dr Green:	Just how old was she?
Mrs Stevens:	She was only seventeen, she had all her life before her.
Dr Green:	That must have been devastating. Can you bear to talk any more about it?
Mrs Stevens:	Yes.
Dr Green:	I should add that you can stop this conversation at any time if it gets too painful.

Assuming that the bereaved person allows the dialogue to continue, there are several areas to be covered. These should include checking whether she was present at the time of death, how she felt at that time, and whether she was able to say goodbye. If she was not able to be present her reactions should be explored, and her reasons for not being there understood.

Dr Green: Were you there when Emily died?

Mrs Stevens: Yes.

Dr Green: How did you feel?

Mrs Stevens: Devastated, I realized there was no way she was going to come back.

Dr Green: Were you able to say goodbye to her?

Mrs Stevens: Yes, that was the good thing: I was able to cuddle her and say goodbye, even though it was awful.

You should next ask her if she saw the individual who died after death, and how she responded. You should be alert to any evidence of avoidance or difficulty in accepting the reality of what had happened.

Dr Green: Were you able to see Emily on any other occasion after that?

Mrs Stevens: Yes, when she was in the Chapel of Rest.

Dr Green: How did she look?

Mrs Stevens: At peace.

Dr Green: How did you feel?

Mrs Stevens: I felt so empty. I realized it was for good; she was not coming back.

It is then important to discuss if she was able to go to the funeral or cremation and how she reacted. It is important to check whether she was able to connect with and express appropriate feelings of grief, as opposed to blocking or suppressing it.

Dr Green: Can you bear to tell me whether Emily was buried or cremated?

Mrs Stevens: She was buried.

Dr Green: Were you able to go to the funeral?

Mrs Stevens: Yes.

Dr Green: And how did you feel?

Mrs Stevens: I couldn't stop crying. Just the thought it was my daughter in that coffin and there was no way back was just almost too awful to contemplate. I cried buckets.

Next you should establish how she fared in the first few weeks after the funeral, and map out the frequency, intensity, nature, and duration of any waves of grief. This will provide an accurate baseline by which to judge further changes. You should also explore if she has felt able to express her feelings of grief in the presence of others, or has been forced to hide them for fear of causing upset.

Dr Green: How did you get on over the next two to three weeks?
Mrs Stevens: It really hit me. I found that from time to time it just hammered me for no reason.
Dr Green: In what way?
Mrs Stevens: I would just be overcome with emotion.
Dr Green: What kind of emotion?
Mrs Stevens: I would feel incredibly lost, despairing, and then very angry.
Dr Green: How often would these feelings hit you?
Mrs Stevens: Oh, many times a day.
Dr Green: Could we try and just map out exactly what happened?
Mrs Stevens: Yes.

It is important to establish how preoccupied she has been with thoughts of the dead person during the waking day and sleep, and whether she has had any dreams or nightmares. The extent of any searching behaviour, sense of presence, illusions, and hallucinations should also be determined.

If the bereaved person is being assessed two to three months after death, it is useful to use the first three weeks as a baseline by which to judge whether or not a slope has developed in respect of waves of grief, searching behaviour, sense of presence, and preoccupation. In normal grief there should be a definite diminution in all of these in the first few months, although it may be a slow process.

When the pattern of grief is abnormal, it is important to check if there are markers, such as were discussed previously.

Thus you should ask if she has been able to accept the reality of the death at an emotional level. What has she done with the belongings, if anything? Is she able to look at photographs? If not, what has she done with them? Has she been able to visit the cemetery or crematorium? If so, how often, and with what impact on her? Is she able to connect with memories of the dead person? Is she describing her daughter in the present or the past tense?

Assessing blocking factors

When the grief is abnormal it is important to explore possible blocking factors. It is worth starting by asking 'What was your relationship with John like?', 'Why do you think you are finding it difficult to come to terms with losing him?', 'What else was happening around the time of his death', 'Were there any particular problems then?', 'Do you believe there is any way in which his death could have been prevented?', 'If so, in what way?', 'Are there particular plans or hopes that you are not going to fulfil as a result?', 'How have other people reacted?', 'How have you felt about the level of support you have been receiving?', and 'Have there been any factors that have made it difficult for you to get in touch with your grief?' These questions will reveal which of the risk factors have been operating.

Counselling

People who have demonstrated a normal pattern of grieving do not need bereavement counselling unless they complain that the slope is taking too long to hit the baseline. Then talking to them in the way already described in 'Assessment' should help them express their grief sufficiently to improve faster and get back to normal life.

Otherwise, counselling should focus on any person who has one or more of those risk factors to any moderate or marked degree. Work by Raphael and others has shown that this reduces the risk of psychiatric morbidity substantially. Such patients benefit from six to eight sessions which focus on helping them connect with and talk through their grief in an active way (Worden 1991).

Some patients with chronic grief may benefit from similar counselling and the use of behavioural techniques like getting them to face photographs and talk about their feelings, or visit the cemetery and talk about their reactions. If chronic grief fails to respond to these simple measures more specialist help is needed from people trained in forced mourning techniques and psychodynamic methods (Worden 1991). specialist cancer nurses, social workers, clinical psychologists, and psychiatrists may have had the necessary training to do this or know someone who has.

Other forms of abnormal grief, like delayed grief, absent grief, oscillating grief, and exploding grief need expert help. Any patient who has developed an anxiety state, a depressive illness, agoraphobia, hypochondriasis, or an alcohol problem should be assessed medically by the General Practitioner or by a psychiatrist. As was discussed earlier in the book, the development of a depressive illness with suicidal ideas, particularly in the context of heavy drinking, necessitates an urgent psychiatric opinion.

When depressive illness is present it is important to treat this first with appropriate antidepressant medication, before beginning any form of counselling. Otherwise, the depression may be intensive and the grief may worsen.

Summary

It is important to distinguish normal from abnormal patterns of grief, and to be able to assess the recently bereaved systematically in order to do this. You should be familiar with the signs and symptoms of the key psychiatric illnesses that can develop after bereavement, and should be aware of those patients who need specialist help rather than simple counselling. The majority of the recently bereaved cope well, and do not need extra help.

References

Brown, G. W. and Harris, T. (1978). *Social origins of depression.* Tavistock, London.

Parkes, C. M. (1965). Bereavement and mental illness I. A clinical study of the grief of bereaved psychiatric patients. *British Journal of Medical Psychology*, **38**, 13–26.

Parkes, C. M., Benjamin, B., and Fitzgerald, R. B. (1969). Broken heart: a statistical study of increased mortality among widows. *British Medical Journal*, **1**, **5635**, 740–3.

Worden, W. J. (1991). *Grief counselling and grief therapy.* Tavistock, London.

12

The psychological costs of caring for cancer patients

The main thrust of this book has been concerned with helping health professionals, and all those involved in caring for cancer patients and their families, to improve their communication skills and their ability to work with people who are often distressed and visibly upset. In this chapter, the needs of the health professionals are considered. 'The cost of caring' has become almost a cliché in health care, but nevertheless it has to be accepted that there is a cost to working effectively with cancer patients and their families, and that this needs to be addressed if individual members of staff are to survive to continue caring at a high level.

It might be argued that the prime consideration in cancer care is the patient and his or her family, and that it is selfish to worry about the professional's personal need for survival. The other side of this argument is that if health carers do not consider their own needs and take some steps to meet them, then they may not be able to go on working in the field. The Americans have a term called 'burn out' that describes the effect of giving to health care to the extent that eventually there is nothing left to give (Maslach 1981; Bernard 1991). The signs of strain leading to 'burn out' are described in Faulkner (1992); but what is important here is that the costs of caring in cancer care are identified and that the factors which can aid the survival of individuals in cancer care are considered.

Participants on workshops described by Maguire and Faulkner (1988) often share their emotional reactions to working with cancer patients and their families, particularly when the prognosis is poor. Among the major feelings identified are those of helplessness, anger, and occasional identification with the patient, and the large emotional problem of dealing with uncertainty and the strong emotions that are engendered in the patient and his or her family.

One of the difficulties for health professionals is their, often strongly held, belief that their main task is to help people who are ill to get better. In cancer care it needs to be accepted that people are not necessarily going to get better, and that some may die relatively quickly. Those who are concerned with palliative care need to know that the most they can give the patient is palliation and the best possible quality of life.

Even those patients who may expect to be cured often have to accept treatment that is very aggressive and causes many problems for the patient and those who care for him or her. A major aid to the survival of the health professional is an acceptance that care can be of good quality and effective without necessarily leading to a cure. Along with this acceptance is the need to know that the inability to offer a cure for cancer for some patients is more to do with the state of the art than it is to do with the personal responsibility of the health professional.

Factors affecting survival
Personal awareness

Most individuals, if asked, would assert that they know themselves: they know their likes, their dislikes, their problem areas. It is suggested here that self-awareness of who one is and where one is coming from in terms of thoughts and beliefs is a very important concept if one is to survive in one's chosen career. Cancer care is not a vocation for everyone, and the important point is to identify whether individuals who have problems in working with cancer patients have those problems because they have not found out enough about themselves as people.

How do we find out about ourselves and gain the insight that will help us survive in the work of our choice? One method is by structured self-analysis. Another method is working with another individual, with a clearly identified structure agreed between both persons. What is being suggested here is not counselling, but may be a part of supervision, with a chance to talk through problems with someone who is trusted and who will help the other individual to gain insight into a particular situation. Whether alone or with an agreed co-worker, personal awareness can grow if particular problems are worked through that have come up in a day's work. For example, individuals may wonder why they felt so helpless in response to a particular patient, or why it was that they felt so suddenly angry when at first glance there seemed no reason to be angry. By reconstructing the situation and looking at the elements of that situation, it should be possible to learn something about the way each of us react in certain circumstances, for example:

Mick: [to colleague] I've had a bad day today. I lost my temper and I just don't know why.

Anna: Why don't you tell me something about it?

Mick:	I don't think I want to. I think it would all blow up again. I'd just rather not say.
Anna:	I think you should try.
Mick:	Well, it was Mr Weston. I've been caring for him as the named nurse ever since he came into the hospice, and when I came back today from my days off, I found that the person who was in charge of him while I was away has organized it so that he's gone home.
Anna:	Who was the other person?
Mick:	It was Lesley, my opposite number. He knew I didn't want that patient to go home.

In the above interaction, it became clear to Mick himself as he opened up and discussed his anger that what he was angry about was not whether or not the patient had gone home, but that he was no longer in control of that patient, and that when he was away, someone else had taken responsibility for 'his' patient. By careful exploration with his colleague he realized that the need to be in control at all times was part of his make-up, and that basically this was to do with something way back in his youth where he had felt in competition with a brother who he felt was more loved than he was. Mick learned through exploring the issues himself that his competition with Lesley, his opposite number, was in fact left over from his youth. Such insight does not always happen; and when it does, people do not necessarily change. What is important is that by his understanding a little more about himself Mick's anger was defused, and he was able to accept, albeit painfully, that this was an area of his make-up that he personally needed to do some work on.

Learning more about one's make-up extends beyond simply understanding why we react in a particular way in a particular situation, and also encompasses our beliefs about life in general and, as was seen in Chapter 10, our own spirituality. This can be a painful business. A nurse, confiding in her tutor that she was having problems in working on a ward with cancer patients, agreed to do some exercises that would perhaps help her to come nearer to understanding the proper nature of her problem. She agreed to look at her own reactions to the patient who was particularly worrying her in situations that arose over an agreed period of time. When she came back to the tutor, she had, by working on her own on the problem, accepted that the patient with whom she was having so much difficulty was someone who reminded her very much of an individual in her own life with whom there had been considerable problems. She said to the tutor, 'You sent me away to find out more about myself. I feel I've done that, but I don't like what I have found.'

The above reaction is not unusual. It is very painful for people to find out that the reasons they have problems in coping in cancer care are in any way to do with what they see as deficits in their own make-up. In fact, everyone has deficits, for the perfect human being does not exist. What is important is for each individual to identify those areas where he or she is prepared to change, and to accept that sometimes, when insight occurs, the resultant decision may not be to change one's make-up, but to change one's job.

Balance

The balance between work and social life is an important factor in surviving in cancer care. The work is demanding in both physical and emotional terms, and it is often easy to spend longer at work than is strictly necessary. This can be a sign of commitment; but it could equally be a sign that the individual has problems, either at work or at home. Similarly, if the imbalance is in favour of social life, it may be that this is one of the first symptoms of 'burn out', in that loss of enthusiasm and an increase in minor illnesses are both signs that the individual is under considerable stress.

Few people have the insight to know when their work gets out of balance with their social life. They almost always need someone to point this out to them, and to be available to discuss any problems which may emerge.

Jenny was a Macmillan nurse who took her work very seriously, and, even though she worked from a clinic, used to give the people she visited her home telephone number. This can be a major cause of imbalance between work and home, in that, if patients have a home number, they will use it. Jenny's moment of truth came when she arrived home from work one night and the telephone was ringing, and she saw stuck on the front of the 'phone a little note that said 'Mum, you have a family.'

What Jenny's daughter was doing was to say 'Please don't keep bringing your work home.' Similarly, at work colleagues may need to have it pointed out that they are coming to work before everybody else and going home after everybody else, and they may need to be confronted with their actions and asked to rethink the way they are operating in the work setting.

An important point in maintaining balance between work and play is to develop personal mechanisms for making a clear break between the two. Travelling home or to work can be a pleasant space in which to wind down from one environment and get ready for the next. Other mechanisms which have been shared on workshops (Maguire and Faulkner 1988) include bathing and changing on arrival home, having a swim between work and going home, using an answerphone at home so there is freedom to collect calls when it is convenient rather than when they arrive, and making a decision not physically to take work home.

Maintaining a balance in activities can be helped considerably by the development of assertiveness skills. This is linked with, but separate from, gaining self-awareness, for people who truly know who they are and where they are coming from usually have little difficulty in saying 'no', because they will have learned their own limitations, what they can do and what would be too much for them to do. Others may feel that it is important always to say 'yes' and to try to do as much as is asked. The difficulty with this is that willing 'slaves' are often over-utilized to a point where they may become too tired to function effectively, and begin to show the signs of 'burn out'.

The importance of saying 'no' is expressed in the reasons for declining an invitation and the way that invitation is declined, for example:

Sister:	Nurse Harris, I'd very much like you to go to Mrs Jones's funeral on Thursday. You were the nurse who did most of the caring while she was with us, and I think it would please the family if you did.
Nurse Harris:	I'm sorry, Sister, I would very much like to have attended the funeral, but in fact it's my day off and I have already made plans.
Sister:	I don't think you understood me, nurse: this is an important part of care for the family, to show that we are with them in this difficult time. I think you had better change your plans, and I can certainly change your day off.
Nurse Harris:	I'm very sorry sister. I would have liked to have gone to the funeral, but it simply isn't possible on this occasion.

In the above exchange, Nurse Harris was being assertive without being aggressive. She gave the sister a clear indication, not only of the fact that she couldn't go to the funeral, but why she could not. Sister tried to change her mind by making her feel selfish; but because Nurse Harris did not feel any guilt about this particular point, having given considerable care to the patient, she was assertively able to make her stand.

Many would argue that this would make Nurse Harris unpopular with the sister, and could in fact affect her leaving report. This fear of sanctions, which may be very real, can affect an individual's ability to be assertive; but in reality, if one looks at successful colleagues, they almost always are people who are assertive in a calm way. They are respected for having clear ideas, providing that they are also showing signs of real care and attention to their patients and their families.

Being assertive may occasionally mean standing up to bullies. Bullies are almost always insecure colleagues who need to be in control and who do not always know how to deal with colleagues who have clear ideas of their own limitations. In this instance, each individual has to make up his or her own mind as to whether they are going to be assertive and maintain their own self-respect, or whether they 'go under' in the name of peace. A very useful book that helps develop assertiveness skills is *When I say 'No' I feel guilty* (Smith 1980).

Preparation

An important question for people to ask in their quest for self-awareness is how well they have been prepared for the job that they are doing, particularly in the area of patient care and communication skills. In a survey of Schools of Nursing in the UK, Faulkner (1985) found that very little time was given to the teaching of communication skills, and that, further, those who taught communication skills did not always feel properly prepared to do this job. The whole issue of the need for training and the way that training can be updated will be considered in Chapter 13.

Organizational issues

Personal survival in cancer care can be affected by organizational issues, and the level of understanding between management and those who are directly responsible for patient care. Good relationships can enhance the working environment, and the responsibility for this is two-way, in that managers need to understand and appreciate the work that clinical staff and others are doing, while those involved in direct care need to understand some of the constraints on their managers. If management issues are openly discussed, then all members of the team should feel that they have the right to give an opinion, and will subsequently feel part of the decision-making rather than that all decisions are made from the top down, sometimes by people who do not fully understand the difficulties in the clinical area.

Working hours

In some hospices all trained staff are part-time, in an attempt to impose balance on those who work in palliative care. In fact, the hours that an individual is able to work while still maintaining balance in life are usually very individual, and will also depend on what responsibilities that individual has outside the work setting. It is argued here that this is an organizational issue that should be discussed with each individual, certainly at the time of appointment to a post, but also subsequently at annual review, in case commitments have changed and the individual concerned requires to change what he or she is doing.

Perhaps more important than the number of hours that are worked is the setting in which those hours are worked. Typically, members of staff work in a particular setting, and expect to stay there; but some areas of cancer care are very draining. In the hospice, for example, in-patient care may involve multiple deaths in a very short time-span. This can be very stressful, and the ability to rotate between the heavier end of cancer care and the more positive end—for example, working in the Day Unit—could give the balance that allows an individual to survive in cancer care for very much longer, even when working full time.

To allow such rotation of staff is obviously more difficult for managers than to leave people in the same setting during the time that they are working. This is particularly true in hospice work, where the Day Care Unit is often organized quite separately from the in-patient unit, and under separate direction. What individuals can do here to help their own survival is to make the case for rotation to their managers, and to come up with creative ideas as to how such a system could work. What is also needed is that other members of staff should be equally happy to rotate, so that when individuals have had a particularly heavy time in their setting there are others who will be prepared to change with them for a short time as a *quid pro quo*.

In hospital, each staff group is generally under the same management, and here it should be possible for individuals to go to their manager and ask to change the specialty that they are in for a period of time. People who need to change would need to use their skills of assertion and give cogent reasons why they need to rotate from the area that they are in. It could be, for example, that a nurse who has been recently bereaved is working in a setting where patients often die. Such a person may need relief from that particular type of nursing, because of the risk of triggering her or his own grief. The change from cancer care to something less demanding should be for a limited time, until the individual in question feels ready to return to his or her own specialty or to take the decision that cancer care is no longer the most appropriate setting to work in.

There is an old adage that says 'a change is as good as a rest', and many health workers would argue that this is true in the working environment; and the standard time set for staying in any one location is five years. It is not always easy, however, to move to a new job. The particular post required may not be available; and there may be family reasons why an individual would wish to stay in the same location. Again, this is a very individual decision that needs to be made in terms of one's own survival and one's ability to continue to give good-quality care. For example, Professor Hancock (Scott 1993) maintains that there is a value and a reward in staying in the same location over a very long period.

Timeout

An alternative to restricting the hours that one works or making decisions on rotation, if that is possible, is that it is sometimes very useful to take time out from the current work situation. In some countries, for example Holland, health-care workers are given a number of free days per year with a variety of titles; but basically these are days in which the individual worker can take time out. This is an area in which considerably more work needs to be done; but it should be possible for any health-care workers who have had a particularly difficult time in their work to ask their managers for a few days off. At present this is only possible if the individual has had a personal bereavement; and, even then, some hospitals demand that the days to go to the funeral and sort out the aftermath of a bereavement should be taken out of annual leave, unless all leave has been used.

In this area, university staff may appear to be more privileged than clinical staff, in that they have the right to take a sabbatical term every few years; but in cancer care the need for timeout could occur much more often than that, though it might only need to be for a few days. In the absence of a managerial policy on time out, it is up to individuals to take the time they can for a break at times of extreme stress. This is difficult, particularly for senior clinical staff, who can easily begin to believe that they are indispensable. Many doctors, for example, in cancer, and particularly in palliative care, even on their days off carry a bleep. This means that they are in fact likely to be working seven days a week. This problem re-emphasizes the importance of learning more about oneself and making clear decisions on space during each working week, and occasionally taking a few extra days and trusting that other members of staff will manage their work very well in the absence of a colleague who needs a break.

This message was brought home very clearly to a nurse manager who was asked to attend two different meetings on the same day. Her own manager responded to her query as to which was the more important meeting by suggesting that she take the day off and not go to either. The nurse responded that she was necessary on both committees, to which her manager replied 'Up and down this country, churchyards are full of indispensable people.'

The concern of the nurse in the above example highlights a major problem with time out, that is, the feeling that in taking time for oneself one is neglecting the duties that one is paid to do. What has to be borne in mind when dealing with this dilemma is the fact that the time out is meant to be therapeutic, and that the individuals who are taking a few days off should come back to their jobs refreshed and more able to give of their best.

Support

The strategies considered so far in this chapter have primarily put the responsibility on individual health-care workers, in that they are encouraged to know more about their own strengths and to consider ways in which they can improve their performances in their current posts. However, no matter how balanced and insightful individuals may be, they may still have their ability to survive in their post affected if there is not support available to them at times of stress. One could argue that each individual bears the responsibility for his or her own level of support; but this can be helped enormously if the organization in which the individual works recognizes the need to support staff and makes, where possible, support mechanisms available for those who wish to use them.

Personal strategies

Faulkner and Maguire (1988) list strategies commonly given by health professionals when asked what strategies they use to gain support against the stress engendered by the emotional demands of clinical practice. Some of these are: unwinding with a partner; going for a long walk; talking to a supportive friend; metaphorically 'kicking the cat'; and outside interests. It can be seen that some of these strategies are more clearly in the area of stress reduction than they are of support; but, nevertheless, health professionals describe them as supportive.

The difficulty with such strategies is that they are not always successful. Supportive friends may not always be available to take the burden of an individual's stress. Partners may have problems of their own, and cats may scratch. Also, these strategies again are seen as the responsibility of the individual who uses them rather than the responsibility of the organization in which that individual works. The problem here is not the strategies, which patently do work for the individuals who describe them, but the fact that many health professionals may still be left with no particular support strategy that will work for them.

It cannot be assumed, for example, that every health-care worker has an understanding partner who will be prepared to listen to the stresses of a demanding post; and often the person who most needs support is the one who is working long hours and not allowing any time for diversional activities.

One can argue that all individuals have stresses in their lives, quite apart from those at work, and therefore have to find their own coping mechanisms for times of stress. Young mothers, for example, often find motherhood very stressful, and many deal with it by linking with other young mothers and sharing the problems of teething and the other responsibilities of child-rearing. Similarly, in cancer care, there are many informal networks in the clinical setting where colleagues take note of each other's stress and provide a sounding-board, maybe over coffee or lunch in the canteen, for the unloading of difficult problems. This informal network can be very successful; but again, may exclude the very people who most need it. Many individuals believe that they have to be seen to be 'tough' and able to cope. Without overall acceptance of the fact that cancer care can be a very stressful occupation, they may feel unable to admit that they themselves need help.

Formal groups

By its very nature, the formal support group gives credence to the notion that support is a vital part of survival for those who work in health care. By setting up formal support groups, those in management are, by definition, giving permission for individuals to admit that sometimes they do need help in managing the stress of working at the sharp end. For a support group to be effective there needs to be a commitment to the group by all who agree to join it and very clear ground rules as to the purpose of the group and how it will work.

Faulkner and Maguire (1988) give basic ground rules for support groups, as follows:

- Confidentiality within the group must be assured. It requires only one group member to gossip outside and trust is lost, as each member wonders who broke faith.
- Problems raised must be professional and relate to work. This avoids embarrassment to those who might disclose highly personal matters in the group but regret it later.
- In parallel with the last point, the group must not be used for personal catharsis.
- The group is not to be used for personal therapy unless this is agreed to be its function by all members and the group is led by a trained psychotherapist.
- The leader must be experienced in group methods and dynamics and be capable of ensuring that discussions are not too superficial or too damaging.
- The leader ensures that no one member monopolizes the group, including herself.

From discussions held at workshops it seems there is some difficulty in the practice of setting up a support group. Very often participants have difficulty in finding a group leader who is not part of the clinical group, and some describe support groups being set up with the unit manager as the group leader. This often causes problems, in that members of the support group are a little cautious of disclosing sensitive material to someone who may write their subsequent report or, indeed, references, if they are looking to move to another post.

Ideally, if one is setting up a formal support group, the leader should come off site, and possibly should be someone who is not a health professional but who has a background in either psychology or psychotherapy. This distance from the group that an outside facilitator represents can be a very strong influence both in engendering trust and encouraging full disclosure of the problems for which an individual may feel the need for support.

If a formal support group is to be started and a facilitator identified, it is probably best if the organization of the group is negotiated at the first meeting. This helps to give participants in the group a sense of ownership and commitment to the parameters that will be set.

The function of a formal support group is to give its individual members a chance to share the problems encountered in clinical practice and also to share feelings and reasons why any particular problem is difficult to cope with. The emphasis should be on generating solutions to the problem in a safe and supportive atmosphere. The function of the leader in this sharing is to facilitate the trust required and to encourage group members to generate potential solutions that any member may choose to try.

A crucial task for the facilitator is to ensure that the group's function is indeed to share problems and seek solutions, and to avoid the group turning into a 'gripe' session where everybody moans about what is going wrong, but then forgets to look for ways in which they might take responsibility for changing those things within their control, and work towards change for things that may need help from higher authority.

The size of the group is important, in that if it is too large it is (a) more difficult to make sure that everybody gets a chance to air his or her problems and (b) people who might be triggered by examples given by others may get their experiences crowded out. The ideal size for a group is between 8 and 12, though much depends on individual facilitators and their feelings about optimum size. Belonging to the group should be something that is totally optional; but there is an inherent risk in not including all members of the unit, in that the group may otherwise come to be seen as a clique or something 'precious'.

Those who do not belong may then become suspicious of the activities of the support group; and for this reason alone, the group should remain open, not only to existing members of staff, but also to people newly joining the staff. Booth and Faulkner (1986) found that a group of tutors became very territorial about their group, and wished to avoid any new members joining because of the impact they might have on the trust of the group.

When the group has been agreed, the facilitator appointed, and the group membership and ground rules formulated, then it is important to set the frequency of meetings of the group and the timing of those meetings. Crucial questions will include whether the group should meet in on- or off-duty time, where it should meet, whether on-site or off-site, and whether the group should have an agenda for its meetings.

It is important in this planning to ensure that all group members have equal opportunity to share their concerns. This may mean having one member of the group given a slot each week at the start of the meeting, followed by other people who have particular and pressing problems. If this type of arrangement is not made clear the potential for one group member to have all the problems is enhanced. Others will then feel that they do not have a chance to identify and share their own problems. This equal opportunity to share is clearly the responsibility of the facilitator, but does require co-operation and understanding from other group members. Finally, it is important when organizing a support group to make time for sharing the positive side of clinical practice, so that the function of the group does not give the overall impression that nothing ever goes right. Once a group is established there may also be humour, as individuals tell stories against themselves, which, with hindsight, have an amusing element. This level of honesty is usually achieved once the group have 'gelled' and are working well together.

Summary

In this chapter it has been seen that caring for cancer patients and their families in an effective way can carry a considerable cost in terms of emotional energy for those who do the caring, and that strategies are required to help individual health-carers to survive, so that they can continue to work with optimum efficiency. It has been argued here that this process can be helped if individuals are aware of their own reactions in their clinical practice, their own beliefs, and how they are affected by patients and their families, their ability to keep the balance between their work and their social life, their potential for being assertive in support of what they believe in, and their preparedness in terms of skills, knowledge, and attitudes to their work.

The effect of organizational issues has been examined, along with the need for support in terms of personal strategies, informal mechanisms, and the potential for formal groups.

References

Bernard, P. (1991). Beyond burn out. *Nursing Standard*, **5** (43), 46–8.

Booth, K. and Faulkner, A. (1986). Problems encountered in setting up support groups in nursing. *Nurse Education Today*, **6**, 244–51.

Faulkner, A. (1985). *Communication in nurse education*. Health Education Council, London.

Faulkner, A. (1992). *Effective interaction with patients*. Churchill Livingstone, Edinburgh.

Faulkner, A. and Maguire, P. (1988). The need for support. *Nursing*, **5** (28), 1010–12.

Maguire, P. and Faulkner, A. (1988). How to improve the counselling skills of doctors and nurses in cancer care. *British Medical Journal*, **297**, 847–9.

Maslach, C. (1981). *Burn out: the cost of caring*. Prentice Hall, Englewood Cliffs, New Jersey.

Scott, I. (1993). Interview with Professor Hancock. *Journal of Cancer Care*, **2** (4), 210–16.

Smith, P. (1980). *When I say 'No' I feel guilty*. Penguin, London.

13

Training in communication skills

The need for training

In the past, conventional medical and nursing curricula have contained little, if any, input on communicating with patients. Faulkner (1985) found that a majority of nurse educators believed that such skills were inherent in health professionals, and there is lively debate in medical schools on whether to include communication as a subject in the curricula. However, when the ability of doctors and nurses to elicit cancer patients' concerns was assessed by asking them to interview simulated patients, recording their interviews, and rating transcripts of audiotapes many were found to be lacking in the behaviours which promote disclosure (Chapter 4). In contrast, behaviours which inhibit disclosure were used more frequently. When the ratio of desired to undesired interviewing behaviours was compared it was found to be one to three. This ratio was not affected by the age of the health professionals, the length of time they had been working with cancer patients, or their professional discipline or training.

Specialist cancer nurses, including Macmillan nurses and health professionals in hospice care, performed no better than other health professionals. Fallowfield and Roberts (1992) have suggested this may be because less than 25 per cent of such nurses have had any formal training in counselling, while many receive no ongoing supervision in their work.

Objective scrutiny, using audiotape recordings of interviews between non-specialist cancer nurses and cancer patients, found that the majority of utterances (over 50 per cent) made by nurses in the study, had the function of blocking patient disclosure (Wilkinson 1991). This was especially true of patients who were being assessed because of recurrent disease (Wilkinson 1991). The ability of the nurses in the study to cover seven key areas (patient's understanding of reason for admission; patient's understanding of diagnosis; history of presenting illness; history of previous illness; physical assessment; social assessment; and psychological assessment) was assessed on 3-point scales (0 = no coverage; 1 = poor coverage; 2 = adequate coverage; 3 = good coverage). Out of a maximum score of 21 the scores for interviews with new patients, those with recurrent disease, and those receiving palliative care were 7.7, 6.0, and 7.1 respectively. Thus nurses were able to retain only a third of the available data, even though they were given sufficient time for their assessment. Moreover, their ability to cover psychological assessment was especially low. Over 60 per cent failed to cover psychological aspects at all, while the rest obtained scores reflecting poor coverage. Even their physical assessments were rated as superficial. Coverage was especially low in patients with recurrent disease, suggesting that nurses were more uncomfortable when assessing these patients. These findings parallel those of Faulkner and Maguire (1984) in a study of nurses caring for mastectomy patients, prior to receiving training in communication skills.

Communicating in other clinical settings
It could be argued that the deficiencies found in health professionals communicating with cancer patients are related to the context of cancer care. However, similar deficits have been found in other clinical settings in both medicine and nursing.

In a systematic assessment of 50 final-year medical students, Maguire and Rutter (1976) found serious deficiencies in their interviewing skills. The students obtained only a third of the data that were available to them, and although only patients who were pleased to co-operate and able to give a coherent history were included, 24 per cent failed to discover the patients' main problems. They most commonly failed to elicit the impact of the presenting problems on the patients' daily lives, mood states, and personal relationships. Few students (22 per cent) clarified the exact nature of the patients' problems, and only 4 per cent were good at responding to patients' cues. Most relied on closed, lengthy, and multiple questions. Many wasted time through needless repetition.

Similar results were found by Faulkner (1980) in a study of 17 student nurses, whose interactions with patients were tape-recorded for later analysis. There was little evidence of effective interactive skills, but all the nurses used blocking tactics and avoidance techniques with patients. As a result, patients had little opportunity to ask questions or disclose concerns. An open questionnaire, using patient vignettes, which was returned by 400 nurses of all grades, suggested similar deficits in the skills and strategies required for effective interaction with patients and their families.

Other studies conducted in London (Macleod Clark 1982), Belfast (Irwin and Bamber 1984), and in Victoria, Australia (Evans *et al.* 1989) have confirmed these deficiencies in key interviewing skills and effective communication. Irwin and Bamber concluded that medical students need most help in the use of clarification, silence, confronting, and picking up cues, and in covering psychological aspects. Faulkner (1980) suggested that nurses should be taught the skills of assessment, but also argued that they had much to unlearn.

Maguire and Rutter (1976) suggested three reasons for these deficiencies: the lack of an explicit model of the areas to be covered in an assessment, and the skills to be used; lack of opportunity to practice interviewing skills under conditions of direct observation but in a safe environment; and the absence of any systematic feedback on performance.

Training in communication skills

There was a need within both medicine and nursing to develop more effective training methods and test their efficacy. Rutter and Maguire (1976) and Maguire *et al.* (1977) evaluated methods which used detailed hand-outs and televised demonstrations, followed by practice under controlled conditions. Those given this training showed significant gains in their interviewing skills compared with students allocated to a control group. However, the exact contribution of feedback on performance to the considerable gains in skills achieved remained unclear.

This was determined by randomizing 48 Manchester medical students to one of four training conditions; the traditional apprenticeship method alone; or that method of teaching plus feedback on interview performance by a tutor, using either a rating scale, or audiotape or videotape feedback (Maguire *et al.* 1978). Students from all three feedback conditions showed significant gains in the amount of information they obtained. However, only the students who had audio or videotape feedback of their performance showed significant gains in their skills. Video appeared to be superior to audiotape feedback in respect of students acquiring the skills of control (keeping patients to the point), avoiding repetition, asking personal questions, and responding to verbal leads. Importantly, students taught only by the traditional apprenticeship method showed no improvement in the amount of information elicited or the skills used.

In nursing, emphasis was laid on the need to make communication an essential part of the nursing curricula and to give tutors the necessary skills to teach. Faulkner and Macleod Clark (1987) describe earlier work (the Communication in Nurse Education project [CINE]) where two nurse tutors were given in-depth training in how to teach communication skills before introducing a programme on effective interaction into six schools of nursing in England. The programme was evaluated using a quasi-experimental design, and two schools of nursing acted as controls.

Teaching methods used included video demonstrations, role play, and audio-feedback. The programme commenced with micro-skills, which were later consolidated by the application of all skills to nursing situations. The findings suggested that the nurses in both the experimental and control groups improved their communication skills overall, but that the nurses in the experimental groups who had had practice and feedback demonstrated substantially greater increments in knowledge and skills than those in the control group. These differences were particularly marked in terms of students' understanding and knowledge of the complexities of communication, and their ability to react appropriately when faced with threatening or emotionally loaded situations.

These immediate benefits of feedback training found in both medicine and nursing have been confirmed by other studies (Irwin and Bamber 1984; Evans *et al.* 1989).

The CINE project had given feedback in groups, but the Manchester work with medical students relied on individual feedback, which was time-consuming for the tutors. Further experiments were conducted to determine if feedback given to medical students within small groups of four students was as effective as individual feedback. This proved to be the case (Roe 1980). These studies also found that the presence of a tutor who understood the content of the skills being taught was necessary for students to feel stretched and make progress. Students who gave themselves or each other feedback in the absence of a tutor made some progress initially, but then showed a marked decline in their skills. Providing feedback of interview performance in small groups became the preferred method of teaching medical students, using audio, rather than video feedback, because of its effectiveness and ease of use. Gask *et al.* (1987, 1988) have since confirmed the value of feedback training of general practice tutors and trainees in small groups.

The work described in both medicine and nursing progressed independently; but similar teaching methods were being developed and evaluated, and similar results emerged. Both were concerned with students, but the CINE project concentrated on general nurses, whereas the Manchester work was developed in the psychiatric clerkship. This raised two important questions: did the medical students retain their skills over time; and, if they did so, did they apply them to patients with non-psychiatric conditions.

A stratified sample of 36 doctors was drawn from those who participated in the Manchester studies as controls or had feedback training, so that the groups were matched for skills before training and time elapsed since training (an average of 5 years, range 4 to 6). Both groups had improved since the psychiatric clerkship; but those given feedback training maintained the superiority on the following skills, clarification, the use of open directive questions, and responding to verbal leads that most promote disclosure. They also showed greater use of key interviewing skills in all patients they interviewed (one with psychiatric illness, one with life-threatening illness and one with chronic disabling illness), but covered psychosocial issues slightly more in their psychiatric patients (Maguire *et al.* 1986).

The ability of trained and control doctors to give patients information and advice was also assessed. Both groups performed poorly, as Faulkner (1980) had found in her study of nurses. Few obtained or took any account of patients' views and expectations. This showed that the learning of skills in eliciting information had not generalized to information-giving. The need to introduce training in information-transfer skills has been acted on in the University of Newcastle, New South Wales (Sanson Fisher *et al.* 1991).

Given the results of the studies described, the time required to provide feedback training can be justified in terms of the short- and longer-term effects of information-eliciting skills.

Training of specialist cancer nurses

These feedback methods were employed in training specialist nurses to monitor and counsel patients undergoing mastectomy. The nurses were given individual feedback of their audiotape assessments of patients about to undergo mastectomy and of patients who had undergone surgery, until they were judged to be clinically competent in the relevant skills and used distancing infrequently.

A group of 152 patients newly diagnosed as having breast cancer and about to undergo mastectomy were randomized to be followed up by these specially trained nurses or to have routine care alone. The nurses provided information, advice, and practical and emotional support before surgery, in the hope that this would prevent psychological and social morbidity. After surgery they visited each patient every two months to monitor their progress (Chapter 5). When patients were found to have problems they were referred to their general practitioner or a back-up psychiatric team.

The doctors and nurses in the control group were able to identify only 15 per cent of those patients who developed psychological and social morbidity, whereas the specially trained nurses were able to recognize 90 per cent of those with problems, and referred 75 per cent of these patients for help. This resulted in a fourfold reduction in psychological and social morbidity in the experimental group 12 to 18 months after surgery when compared with the control group.

The nurses were able to maintain this level of performance providing they had regular supervision and rapid access to the back-up psychiatric team when they encountered particularly difficult situations (Maguire *et al.* 1980, 1983).

Limited intervention

This method of providing counselling and monitoring, which involved two monthly home visits for each patient, meant that the specialist cancer nurses spent a considerable amount of time assessing patients who were coping well. This resulted in an accumulating load, with the attendant risk that those patients who were coping well could become more anxious because they were reminded about their cancer and treatment. The scheme also put the responsibility for psychological care on specialist nurses, and there were complaints from the ward and community staff that they were not being allowed to contribute as much as they would like. Social workers in particular felt that their role was threatened.

A further study was carried out, which sought to compare three conditions. These included the original full monitoring scheme, a limited scheme, and a ward/community scheme. In the limited scheme the specialist nurse was limited to one post-discharge assessment, which was carried out within two months in the patient's home. The aim of this home visit was to carry out an assessment of the patient's physical, social, and psychological adjustment. If any problems were found at that point they were referred either to the general practitioner or the psychiatric back-up team for help. If no problems were found the onus was put on the patient to contact the nurse later if any difficulties developed.

In the ward/community arm the ward nurses were given feedback training and then the district nurse or health visitor to whom the patient was discharged was offered similar training.

A randomized controlled trial was carried out to assess the impact of these interventions. Importantly, the limited intervention arm proved as effective as the full intervention arm (Wilkinson *et al.* 1988). However, the ward/community arm did not prove as effective as had been hoped. The ward nurses became committed to improving skills and showed a clear increase in their assessment skills following feedback training. They did not however all achieve clinical competence in psychological assessment, particularly the assessment of anxiety and depression, where they were nervous of making errors. The training was less effective with the district nurses and health visitors, who seemed poorly motivated to improve their interviewing and assessment skills.

The differences between the ward and the community staff were largely explained in terms of group dynamics, in that all trained staff on the ward were very involved and became a very cohesive group. When the community nurses were involved, it was usually one nurse in any of the health centres involved. Consequently, these nurses were often teased by colleagues not involved in the study (Faulkner 1984), and felt isolated.

The study confirmed that specialist nurses who were willing to learn and apply the key skills, particularly within the full and limited intervention arms (Wilkinson *et al.* 1988), were able to recognize and refer patients who developed problems or carry out counselling themselves; but all specialist nurses were not comfortable in this role. The training had a subsequently beneficial effect on the level of psychosocial morbidity. But a major question about training remained. How could the large numbers of health professionals involved in cancer care, whether in cancer hospitals, hospices, general hospitals, or the community, be helped to acquire these skills and relinquish ineffective behaviours and distancing strategies?

Development of workshops

The first workshops were initiated by the Royal College of Nursing (RCN), and were for cancer nurses only. They were of three days' duration, residential, and limited to 24 participants. Teaching methods included exercises in dyads and triads, video demonstration, and role play (Faulkner and Nurse 1981). The courses were positively evaluated, but two areas caused concern. Firstly, nurses reported feeling 'diminished' by the dyad and triad exercises, but also threatened if emotionally loaded material was discussed in the absence of a tutor. Secondly, the tutors were concerned that the nurses 'alibied' their deficits in skilled behaviour by scapegoating doctors.

The workshops took place at Hollyroyde College, through the Extra-Mural Department of Manchester University. When the RCN courses were withdrawn as part of changes in their education policy, new courses were developed, which were to be of three to five days' duration, with two-day follow-up after six months. They were planned to be multi-disciplinary, residential, and voluntary, and would use learner-centred methods of teaching/facilitation (Maguire and Faulkner 1988).

Each workshop of 16 to 20 participants began with the two facilitators inviting the participants to meet in two small groups to set their own agenda. They were asked to identify which communication situations they had found most difficult to cope with in recent months in three areas of their experiences: communication with patients; communicating with relatives; and communicating with colleagues. It was emphasized that they should base their problem list on real situations they had encountered, rather than on theoretical issues. This exercise was carried out to highlight the importance of obtaining an accurate problem list from an individual before beginning any counselling.

The participants next met in a plenary session to report back their agenda. As in real life, they usually reported more problems than could be dealt with in the time available. So they were asked to put them in order of priority. A score of '0' meant that the participants considered they already had the skill or that the situation was not relevant to them. A score of 10 meant it was imperative that they practised it because of its relevance and/or their lack of confidence in handling it. An intermediate score reflected the salience to them of the item. The scores on each item were then summed and ranked in order from the highest score to the lowest score. The top agenda items then represented the workshop consensus about the priorities to be covered. A typical agenda is shown in Table 13.1.

Learning methods
In the light of the experience gained in training medical and nursing students, general practitioners, and specialist cancer nurses, and the experiences in the RCN workshops, two particular methods were emphasized. First, the content of an assessment interview and the key skills were made explicit through the use of demonstration videotapes. How and how not to handle certain difficult situations were also demonstrated on videotape. And second, participants were given an opportunity to practise key communication tasks in small groups, and

Table 13.1 Top ten items on a typical agenda

		% of maximum
1. Managing uncertainty	197	94
2. Basic assessment	187	89
3. Handling anger	179	85
4. Multiple losses	161	77
5. Psychiatric disorder	151	72
6. Confronting colleagues	149	71
7. Handling denial	148	70
8. Supporting relative when prognosis is poor	140	67
9. Discussing nurses' attitudes to abusive patients	131	62
10. Non-compliant patients	124	59

Note: 21 participants—maximum possible score + 210.

andwere given feedback on their performance. The key method used is that of role play.

Role play

The value of role play is that it both allows participants to play the part of the particular patient, relative, or colleague with whom they have experienced difficulty, and also allows the practice of key tasks in their own role as doctor or nurse, social worker or chaplain. The level of complexity of the role play can be controlled by starting with simpler situations before moving on to more difficult ones. This minimizes the risk of de-skilling the participants, who come to realize that their skills are not at the level that they may have assumed they were before the workshop. Most participants are unaware of the extent to which they use distancing strategies as a defence against the patient's emotional pain.

Clear ground rules are negotiated to minimize de-skilling further. These include the use of 'time-out'. By definition, if health professionals volunteer to deal with a difficult situation because they want help with it they are bound to get stuck in the role play that parallels that situation. So they are encouraged to call time-out when they become stuck, or otherwise the facilitator will stop the role play immediately. The group are given the responsibility of helping the health professional move the interview forward by suggesting alternative strategies that might help him or her. Thus the activity then becomes a shared one, rather than leaving the health professional feeling it is just he or she who is 'in the hot seat'. Moreover, the group are invited to offer positive comments first, before being allowed to make any constructive criticisms. When they make constructive criticisms they are asked to suggest possible strategies that might be used.

When the group have offered a number of strategies the interviewers are invited to decide which one they wish to use and test out. They can be given validation about its effect by asking the group for comments about how it went subsequently. The health professional playing the part of the patient or relative can also provide valuable feedback. In this way the participants come to realize that particular behaviours have positive outcomes, while other behaviours inhibit patients' or relatives' disclosure and may heighten their distress.

In setting up such role play it is crucial for the tutor to make it personally safe for the interviewer and the role player. Thus, the people playing the parts of the patient or the relative should be asked to check whether they are comfortable playing that part, or whether it is too close to some real-life experience that caused them anguish. If there is any risk of triggering they should be dissuaded from taking the part. Similarly, if interviewers elect to take on a particularly difficult situation it is important to check that they are not going to be overwhelmed by it in the light of some recent experience. This screening makes role play 'safe', in that the facilitator will not leave any player in a role if such 'triggering' occurs or real distress ensues.

Impact of workshops

Each workshop was informally evaluated, and invariably positively. Although such enthusiasm was rewarding, it did not indicate whether (a) teaching methods were valid, or (b) the actual skills of the participants improved and were maintained over time.

To examine these questions, we developed a project, funded by the Cancer Research Campaign (CRC), to evaluate the effects of the workshops, using a pre-, and post-test design, and involving over 200 participants, including doctors, nurses, social workers, and a few members of the clergy.

Each participant was asked to assess a simulated patient at the beginning and end of the workshop, and at the follow-up days six months later. These interviews were audiotaped for later analysis, and rated using a scale developed by Booth *et al.* (Faulkner 1992). Positive changes had occurred in most of the desired skills, while the workshops had helped the participants relinquish most of their ineffective behaviours. Follow-up data suggest that most skills remained at a significantly higher level than before training, though there had been some decline. In the absence of a control group it could be argued that these gains represent a practice effect. A quasi-experimental study was carried out to test for this with participants from four further workshops. In two of these workshops the participants were randomized to either assessment interviews at the beginning *and* end of the workshop, or at the end of the workshop only. In one, assessment interviews were conducted at the beginning of the workshop, and in the other, at the end only. A practice effect was not shown; but, as in the larger study, significant improvements were found in the desired behaviours, while the use of the inhibitory behaviours was substantially reduced.

Application of learning

From the participants' feedback at follow-up it was clear that the application of the skills they had learned was often problematic within the context of their daily work. Some found it difficult to integrate this new learning into their prior mode of assessment and communication. Others found it difficult because they felt they did not get the necessary support for this way of working from colleagues or supervisors. This supports the findings of Faulkner's (1984) work with community nurses, and that of Wilkinson (1991) with cancer nurses. The availability of psychological and psychiatric back-up for those patients requiring special help was also seen as a necessary component if people are to maintain and apply their learning.

The workshops are essentially skills-based, but do devote a mandatory session to the issues of how health professionals can work in this way and survive emotionally. The approach of Razavi *et al.* (1988) to training was different, in that it focused on attitudes towards 'death and dying' and helping health professionals cope better with terminally ill patients and their relatives. A semantic differential questionnaire was used to assess changes in the participants' attitudes towards illness and death. The authors found that their workshops achieved a significant change in attitudes for those allocated to training compared with those in a control group. Subjects reporting more negative attitudes at the beginning of the training benefited most.

A key issue for future initiatives is the extent to which training should concentrate on skills versus attitudes and feelings. Further work is required to clarify this issue.

Self-assessment

Health professionals who are motivated to improve their skills could after brief training assess their own performance using audiotape or videotape and then systematically assess whether or not they have the key skills. This self-monitoring can ensure that effective practice does not lapse over time.

Skills that are particularly worth assessing include establishing eye-contact at the outset of the interview; being able to clarify the patient's concerns; and responding to cues, particularly verbal cues about emotional distress. Being willing to ask questions with a psychological content and to show interest in the home situation as well as making supportive comments also make it more likely that the patient will reveal any underlying concerns and distress (Marks *et al.* 1979). Keeping the patient to the point and being able to maintain reasonable eye-contact while taking notes are also important skills.

Doctors who are effective at eliciting patient concerns and distress do so by increasing the number and rate of cues given by the patient about possible problem areas. This cue emission is increased, as discussed in Chapter 4, by the use of open directive questions with a psychological focus, by clarifying verbal cues given by the patient, and by the use of empathy (Goldberg *et al.* 1993).

Health professionals could establish a checklist of these behaviours and determine the extent to which they are using or not using them, with occasional support from a colleague or supervisor.

Other behaviours that increase disclosure and can be monitored include summarizing what the patient has said, and checking the accuracy of understanding by the use of understanding hypotheses (educated guesses).

Such a checklist should also include the negative behaviours highlighted in Chapter 4. These include the use of premature advice and premature reassurance, closed questions, and time spent on clarifying physical concerns.

Most patients and relatives will agree to the use of a small tape-recorder providing it is explained that this is to help improve the health professional's ability to communicate, and that the recording is confidential. However well workshops or such self-assessment help individuals improve their skills in the short term, it is likely that ongoing training and supervision will be necessary to ensure proper integration of these skills into the health professional's day-to-day work.

This might best be achieved by distance learning in which, after an initial residential workshop, individuals send their tapes to be rated and are given detailed feedback over a period of time. This approach is currently being tested at Trent Palliative Care Centre following day-release courses and the Cancer Research Campaign Psychological Medicine Group have also been exploring the use of distance learning. Alternatively, it might be achieved through ongoing small-group supervision. Such training will only be possible if a pool of teachers can be recruited and trained.

Training the teachers

A major barrier to the implementation of training in interviewing skills and communication within the cancer field is the lack of appropriate teachers. A major question is how health professionals can best be prepared for this role.

As a result of the poor communication skills found in student nurses, the Health Education Council funded a survey to determine the place of communication teaching in the curricula. A survey, addressed to all tutors involved in teaching communication skills, elicited a 75 per cent return (Faulkner 1985). The results of the study suggested that less than 5 per cent of tutors felt that they had adequate preparation to teach the subject, while the Directors of Nurse Education put the figure at 2 per cent.

Both directors of nursing and tutors felt that it was very important to teach communication skills (87 per cent; 95 per cent), but only 5 per cent of the curriculum time was thought to be given to the subject. Perhaps the most important finding from the survey was the perceived lack of courses available for tutors to attend in order to improve their ability to teach communication skills.

Training methods

It has been found that didactic modes of training clinical teachers to teach interviewing skills are less effective than experiential modes, in which the teachers first experience the methods of interview training themselves before they teach the interviewing skills. Teachers who have had the feedback training themselves not only show more improvement in their own skills, but are also more aware of their own strengths and weaknesses, and are more sensitive to their students' needs and reactions (Naji *et al.* 1987).

This finding is supported by the results of the CINE Phase II project (Faulkner and Macleod Clark 1987), which concentrated on teaching nurse-tutor students how to use experiential methods in teaching communication skills. Two colleges, where tutor-training programmes are offered, co-operated in the study, which was evaluated, for the whole of one academic year, and one of these incorporated this approach in the curricula for subsequent courses. Tutors who were followed up after the course were found to use experiential methods more than those who had not had the training.

Workshops have been implemented which seek to help those who wish to teach. Participants attend the workshops on assessment, interviewing, and counselling skills already described. They then attend a second workshop which focuses on practising teaching methods. Efforts have been made to select at least two people from each institution to participate in these workshops, in the hope that they will be able to give each other support and co-facilitate similar workshops (Faulkner *et al.* 1991). As a result of this initiative, the pairs of tutors suggested that they required support and updating in order to develop and run courses effectively. Help the Hospices are currently funding a support programme for these tutors, who meet twice a year for two days with two facilitators. A North and South group has been established, with a core group of five pairs in each group. Other pairs of tutors attend when possible. To date, informal evaluation suggests that the support has had a positive effect, especially in terms of improved teaching skills and personal growth. The impact on teaching skills and on the students taught by these teachers has yet to be evaluated objectively.

The American Academy on Physician and Patient has mounted a major initiative in the teaching of interviewing skills within medicine in general. Their week-long workshops seek to help participants improve both their interviewing and teaching skills (Bird *et al.* 1993). Equal attention is paid in the agenda to skills work and to personal awareness, attitudes, and feelings. The skills work is practised in small groups of 4, while the personal awareness work takes place in groups of 8. The impact of these workshops has yet to be evaluated.

Training in the workplace

The optimal way to help health professionals improve their interviewing, assessment, and communication skills would be to provide them with ongoing feedback training and supervision within their work setting. This should ensure that problems in integrating and applying their skills within a clinical practice could be overcome. Such training will only be feasible if senior medical, nursing, and social work staff are trained in these skills and in effective teaching methods. They could then initiate ongoing training with their junior staff.

Yet most work in the field of teaching communication skills has focused on medical and nursing students, junior doctors, and nurses. An exception to this is the work described by Maguire and Faulkner (1988), where many participants are relatively senior. Initiatives are also being mounted to assess the impact of training senior staff and to see how this training affects junior staff.

It would be easier to emphasize the importance of training in these skills if there were more solid evidence about the actual impact of doctors' and nurses' use of key skills on the patient's psychological adaptation to diagnosis and treatment and the level of social and psychological morbidity. More research is needed to demonstrate this.

Competencies of specialist nurses

As a minimum, specialist nurses ought to be proficient in the skills that promote disclosure that were discussed in Chapter 4, and should have been able to relinquish distancing strategies and the negative behaviours that inhibit disclosure. They should be able to handle a variety of difficult situations that they encounter commonly, such as dealing with an angry or distressed patient, handling collusion and the other situations discussed in the chapters on dealing with difficult situations, and handling conflict.

They should be familiar with at least one validated model of counselling, and be able to apply it in practice, while recognizing their own limitations and indications for referral to other health professionals. They should be able to identify patients with an anxiety state, a depressive illness, a body-image problem, sexual difficulties, or interpersonal problems. They should also be able to distinguish normal from abnormal grief, and be aware which patients might need referral for more specialist help.

They should be aware of signs of over-involvement or over-identification with patients, and be familiar with the concepts of transference and counter-transference. They should be comfortable with empowering patients rather than trying to act for them. They should be encouraged to continue their education, evolve their own working methods, and accept ongoing supervision, as well as to scrutinize their time-management.

They should also be aware of ethical issues concerning the treatment of cancer and randomized control trials.

In addition to these basic skills and the ability to deal with difficult situations, they should try to ensure that they become competent in the skills of anxiety-management training and cognitive therapy. It would also help if they possessed the necessary teaching skills to help other professionals upgrade their communication skills.

They should be able to audit the pattern of their work in order to determine if they are being unduly selective in terms of the kinds of patients they are seeing, whether in terms of cancer site, ethnic group, age, or any other factor.

Summary

The skills that will help health professionals improve their ability to elicit cancer patients' concerns have been identified. Effective methods of training have been developed. However, the majority of health professionals involved in cancer care have yet to receive training in basic assessment skills and how to deal with more difficult situations or actual counselling methods. Important initiatives have been mounted to try to overcome these difficulties; but much depends on improving the skills of those responsible for teaching, especially in the area of experiential and interactive teaching.

References

Bird, J., Hall, A., Maguire, P., and Heavy, A. (1993). Workshops for consultants on the teaching of clinical communical skills. *Medical Education*, **27**, 181–5.

Evans, B. J., Stanley, R. O., Bowers, G. D., and Sweet, B. (1989). Lectures and skills workshops as teaching formats in a history taking course for medical students. *Medical Education*, **23**, 364–70.

Fallowfield, L. and Roberts, R. (1992). Cancer counselling in the United Kingdom. *Psychology and Health*, **6**, 107–17.

Faulkner, A. (1980). The student nurse's role in giving information to patients. Steinberg Collection, RCN, London.

Faulkner, A. (1984). Teaching non-specialist nurses assessment skills in the aftercare of mastectomy patients. Steinberg Collection, RCN, London.

Faulkner, A. (1985) *Communication in nurse education. A survey of schools of nursing*. Health Education Council, London.

Faulkner, A. (1992). The evaluation of training programmes for communication skills in palliative care. *Journal of Cancer Care*, **1**, 75–8.

Faulkner, A. and Macleod Clark, J. (1987). Communication skills teaching in nurse education. In *Nursing education: research and developments* (ed. B. Davis), pp. 189–205. Croom Helm, London.

Faulkner, A. and Maguire, P. (1984). Teaching ward nurses to monitor cancer patients. *Clinical Oncology*, **10**, 383–9.

Faulkner, A. and Nurse, G. (1981). Counselling cancer patients. *Nursing Focus*, **2** (8), 268–9.

Faulkner, A., Webb, P., and Maguire, P. (1991). Communication and counselling skills: educating health professionals working in cancer and palliative care. *Patient Education and Counselling*, **18**, 3–7.

Gask, L., McGrath, G., Goldberg, D., and Millar, T. (1987). Improving the psychiatric skills of established general practitioners: evaluation of group teaching. *Medical Education*, **21**, 362–82.

Gask, L., Goldberg, D., Lesser, A. L., and Millar, T. (1988). Improving the psychiatric skills of the general practice trainee: the evaluation of a group training course. *Medical Education*, **22**, 132–8.

Goldberg, D. P., Jenkins, L., Millar, T., and Faragher, E. B. (1993). The ability of training general practitioners to identify psychological distress among their patients. *Psychological Medicine*, **23**, 183–93.

Irwin, W. G. and Bamber, J. H. (1984). The evaluation of medical student behaviours in communication. *Medical Education*, **18**, 90–5.

Macleod Clark, J. (1982). Nurse–patient verbal interaction. Steinberg collection, RCN, London.

Maguire, P. and Faulkner, A. (1988). How to do it: improve the counselling skills of doctors and nurses in cancer care. *British Medical Journal*, **297**, 847–9.

Maguire, G. P. and Rutter, E. R. (1976). History taking for medical students. 1—Deficiencies in performance. *Lancet*, **ii**, 556–8.

Maguire, G. P., Clark, D., and Jolly, B. (1977). An experimental comparison of three courses in history taking skills for medical students. *Medical Education*, **11**, 175–82.

Maguire, G. P., Roe, P., Goldberg, D., Jones, S., Hyde, C., and O'Dowd, T. (1978). The value of feedback in teaching interviewing skills to medical students. *Psychological Medicine*, **8**, 695–704.

Maguire, P., Tait, A., Brooke, M., Thomas, C., and Sellwood, R. (1980). The effect of counselling on the psychiatric morbidity associated with mastectomy. *British Medical Journal*, **281**, 1454–6.

Maguire, P., Brooke, M., Tait, A., Thomas, C., and Sellwood, R. (1983). The effect of counselling on physical disability and social recovery after mastectomy. *Clinical Oncology*, **9**, 319–24.

Maguire, P., Fairbairn, S., and Fletcher, C. (1986). Consultation skills of young doctors: 1—Benefits of feedback training in interviewing as students persist. 2—Most young doctors are bad at giving information. *British Medical Journal*, **292**, 1573–8.

Marks, J., Goldberg, D., and Hillier, V. (1979). Determinants of general practitioners to detect psychiatric illness. *Psychological Medicine*, **9**, 337–53.

Naji, S., Maguire, P., Fairbairn, S. A., Goldberg, D. P., and Faragher, E. B. (1987). Training clinical teachers in psychiatry to teach interviewing skills to medical students. *Medical Education*, **20**, 140–7.

Razavi, D., Delvaux, N., Farvacques, C., and Robaye, E. (1988). Immediate effectiveness of brief psychological training for health professionals dealing with terminally ill cancer patients: a controlled study. *Social Sciences and Medicine*, **27**, 369–75.

Roe, E. (1980). Training medical students in interviewing skills. MSc thesis, University of Manchester.

Rutter, D. R. and Maguire, G. P. (1976). History taking for medical students. II—Evaluation of a training programme. *Lancet*, **ii**, 558–60.

Sanson-Fisher, R. W., Redman, S., Walsh, R., Mitchell, K., Reid, A. L. A., and Perkins, J. J. (1991). Training medical practitioners in information transfer skills: their new challenge. *Medical Education*, **25**, 322–3.

Wilkinson, S. (1991). Factors which influence how nurses communicate with cancer patients. *Journal of Advanced Nursing Studies*, **16**, 677–88.

Wilkinson, S., Maguire, P., and Tait, A. (1988). Life after breast cancer. *Nursing Times*, **84** (40), 34–7.

14

Training resources available

Learning opportunities

There are many courses to help individuals improve their communication skills and develop the ability to take on a counselling role. Some universities, for example, offer a diploma in counselling, which can be taken full or part-time. Others offer a basic degree in communication, which covers both theory and practice.

With the move to semesters rather than terms, and courses which can be taken module by module to accumulate enough credits for a degree, it is possible to register for modules of choice. Sheffield University, for example, offers a Diploma/MSc in Palliative Care which includes a module on communication and one on bereavement that can be studied as discrete units.

The overriding problem for many health professionals is time and access to programmes of study. Also, many courses are not directly related to health care. It was seen in Chapter 13 that short, focused workshops improve the skills of the participants, and that those skills are generally maintained over time. Workshops, based on the model described in this book, are listed below:

1. Communication and counselling skills

(Open to all health professionals involved in cancer and palliative care.)

Five days, with 2-day follow-up after 6 months

Help the Hospices offer these courses twice a year. These workshops are designed for doctors, nurses, and other health professionals who are working with terminally ill and cancer patients. The sessions focus on helping to develop further the ability to assess and counsel patients and relatives, and to deal with psychological and social aspects of care. Workshops include demonstrations, discussions, practice, and feedback.

Such is the intense nature of the work that numbers of participants are limited. Details from: Help the Hospices, 34–44 Britannia Street, London WC1X 9JG.

Three days, with 2-day follow-up after 6 months

These courses are similar to the above, but suitable for those who cannot take five days away from work. They are offered collaboratively by Help the Hospices and the Extra-Mural Department of the University of Manchester, in response to the demand from health professionals.

Details from: Lyn Palethorpe, Department of Extra-Mural Studies, University of Manchester, M13 9PL.

Three days

The Cancer Research Campaign Psychological Medicine Group (Manchester) offer these workshops on counselling skills which cater for individuals' learning needs. The majority of the time is spent in small-group work. This allows considerable opportunity for participants to practise key skills and receive individual feedback on their performance. Detailed workbooks are provided.

Details from: Mrs Sue Moore, CRC Psychological Medicine Group, Stanley House, Christie Hospital, Wilmslow Road, Manchester M20 9BX.

Three days (for senior clinicians who work predominantly with patients with cancer)

The Cancer Research Campaign Communication and Counselling Research Centre offer these workshops, which are based on a model pioneered in the United States. There are a maximum of four participants per tutor, and participants are given constructive feedback on their skills together with experience in teaching junior staff to improve their skills.

Details from: Dr Lesley Fallowfield, CRC Communication and Counselling Research Centre, London Hospital Medical College, Turner Street, London E1 2AD.

2. Workshops on bereavement

(Open to all health professionals involved in working with bereaved individuals.)

Three days, plus two-day follow-up
These courses are offered collaboratively by Help the Hospices and the
Extra-Mural Department of the University of Manchester. The course
content is learner-centred, with considerable small-group work to help
participants improve their skills in identifying those individuals who can
cope with their grief within their own social circle, those who need some
help, and those who need referral. Participants are encouraged to
determine their personal limits and to set boundaries.

Details from: Lyn Palethorpe, Extra-Mural Department, University of
Manchester, Manchester M13 9PL.

**3. Courses for those wishing to teach communication and
counselling skills in cancer and palliative care**
Three days, plus two-day follow-up
Help the Hospices offer these courses twice a year. They are open to
health professionals who have completed a skills-based workshop, and
are learner-centred. Content includes course-planning and budgeting,
teaching methods (including role play, sculpting, and the use of videotapes), and potential problem areas.

Details from: Help the Hospices, 34–44 Britannia Street, London
WC1X 9JG.

Three days
The Cancer Research Campaign Psychological Medicine Group
(Manchester) offer small but intense workshops which are limited to
eight participants, and seek to help experienced health professionals
learn how to use video and role play in order to teach communication
and counselling skills.

General workshops for teachers
American Academy on Physician and Patient
This American group run five-day workshops designed to help
experienced health professionals improve their own interviewing and
teaching skills. They include skill-based work, lectures, and personal
awareness groups.

Details can be obtained from: Penny Williamson, 4611 Keswick
Road, Baltimore, MD 21210, USA.

The Medical Interview Teaching Association—Workshops
This group hold annual workshops for teachers within Great Britain. Facilitators come from both Great Britain and the United States. They follow the American Academy model in combining both skill-based and personal awareness work.

Details can be obtained from: Angela Hall, CRC Communication and Counselling Research Centre, London Hospital Medical College, Turner Street, London E1 2AD.

Further details of short courses for those involved in Cancer and Palliative care can be obtained from:

St Christopher's Hospice Information Service, 51–59 Lawrie Park Road, Sydenham, London SE26 6DZ.

Education Department, Cancer Relief Macmillan Fund, 15/19 Britten Street, London SW3 3TZ.

Help the Hospices, 34–44 Britannia Street, London WC1X 9JG.

Education Department, Marie Curie Cancer Care, 28 Belgrave Square, London SW1X 8QG.

Information Manager, Trent Palliative Care Centre, Sykes House, Little Common Lane, Sheffield S11 9NE.

Videotapes
Videotapes are a potent resource for teaching communication and counselling skills. The following are based on the model illustrated in this book:

Set of 5 (Help the Hospices)
1. Assessing a dying patient
This videotape shows the skills of assessment, which are illustrated by an interview with a female patient who is dying of cancer.

Part 1:   Doctor–patient physical assessment

Part 2:   Nurse–patient psychological assessment

2. Breaking collusion
The difficult area of sharing the truth when a couple wish to protect each other is addressed in this videotape.

Part 1:   Doctor interviews wife of patient to elicit her concerns
                 re husband's prognosis.

Part 2:   Doctor interviews husband to assess his awareness of
               diagnosis/prognosis.

Part 3:   Doctor interviews couple together to facilitate sharing
               of awareness.

3. The difficult patient

Patients are occasionally described as 'difficult' or 'withdrawn' when
they may in fact be simply unhappy. This videotape shows both
effective and ineffective ways to attempt to persuade a patient to share
his or her problems.

Part 1:   Ineffective interview, with nurse blaming patient for
               being uncooperative.

Part 2:   More effective interview, where nurse attempts to see
               patient's perspective on problems.

4. The young, angry patient

This videotape shows a young woman, dying of cancer, who is trying to
make sense of her current situation. Both ineffective and effective
interview techniques are demonstrated.

Part 1:   Doctors shows ineffective techniques of interviewing
               with resultant anger on part of patient.

Part 2:   Effective doctor/patient interview where patient feels
               safe enough to air concerns and make decisions about
               future treatment.

5. Advocacy

The nurse often finds herself in the role of patient's advocate against the
doctor who may have a different perception of a problem. This
videotape shows both ineffective and effective advocacy.

Part 1:   Doctor/nurse battle showing how advocacy can turn
               into a win–lose situation for both professionals.

Part 2:   Effective advocacy where nurse uses knowledge and
               understanding to put patient's case to doctor.

Note

Each videotape is accompanied by full teaching notes and suggestions
for group discussions.

Details available from: Ann Faulkner, Deputy Director, Trent Palliative Care Centre, Sykes House, Little Common Lane, Sheffield S11 9NE.

Set of 4

1. Confronting a colleague

Health professionals often find it difficult to confront a colleague with inappropriate or unprofessional behaviour. This videotape shows ineffective and effective ways of confronting a colleague.

Part 1:   The doctor attempts to discipline a nurse who appears to be making mistakes on the ward.

Part 2:   The doctor attempts to make sense of a change in the behaviour of a nurse.

2. Sequencing

An important part of assessment is to encourage the individual to complete each sequence of an event before moving on. This video demonstrates how an assessment can given inaccurate information if sequences are interrupted.

Part 1:   The nurse makes assumptions on the patients' problems and offers inappropriate advice.

Part 2:   The nurse encourages the patient to complete each sequence before 'moving on' and gains a more accurate assessment of current problems.

3. Helping a patient to discuss her concerns with a partner

Even in a close and loving relationship, patients and their loved ones may find it difficult to discuss a fear-provoking diagnosis and prognosis. In this videotape, the doctor helps the patient to explore some of these issues.

Part 1:   The doctor offers inappropriate advice.

Part 2:   The doctor explores the situation from the patient's point of view and helps her make appropriate decisions.

Part 3:   The doctor helps the patient plan strategies for talking to her partner.

4. *Assessing a bereaved individual*

Most bereaved individuals work through their grief with the help of their own social circle. This videotape shows an assessment interview eight weeks after a death to identify if individuals are coping with their grief or need further help.

Note
Each videotape is accompanied by a full transcript and suggested questions for group discussion.

Details available from: Ann Faulkner, Deputy Director, Trent Palliative Care Centre, Sykes House, Little Common Lane, Sheffield S11 9NE.

Child of a dying parent

Pam is dying of breast cancer. Her husband, Rob, has deliberately withheld from their children, Duncan (12) and Christopher (14), the true nature of their mother's illness. This he believes is to protect them, and to protect their mother.

Professor Ann Faulkner negotiates access to the children, and then explores with Duncan and Christopher their feelings and reactions to their mother's illness and death.

This video is produced as a teaching aid for those working with dying patients and their relatives, and with the bereaved. It is produced to the highest quality, and comes complete with teaching notes. It has been awarded a British Medical Association certificate of educational merit.

Details available from: Ann Faulkner, Deputy Director, Trent Palliative Care Centre, Sykes House, Little Common Lane, Sheffield S11 9NE.

Linkward series: Why won't they talk to me?—by Rob Buckman and Peter Maguire

This series include five tapes which illustrate common pitfalls in communicating with cancer patients and their relatives, and suggest possible solutions. Topics include use of distancing strategies, breaking bad news, dealing with anger, and checking patient awareness.

Details available from: Linkward Productions, Post 63, Shepperton Studio Centre, Squiresbridge Road, Shepperton, Middlesex, TW17 0QD.

Pfizer series: Breaking bad news
These three videotapes are produced by Pfizer to help doctors to improve their skills in handling bad news situations. Professor Ann Faulkner demonstrates breaking bad news to a patient, a relative, and parents, and discusses the issues surrounding each encounter. They have been awarded a British Medical Association Bronze award.
Available from: Pfizer, Sandwich, Kent, CT13 9NJ.

Books
Two publications are available which are based on the research and model described in earlier chapters of this book.

Faulkner, A. (1992). *Effective interaction with patients.* Churchill Livingstone, Edinburgh. (Translated into French and Swedish.)

Faulkner, A. (1993). *Teaching effective interaction in health care.* Chapman and Hall, London.

INDEX